Unlossable Love
(No Matter How Hard You Try)

JOHN BOYANOWSKI AND BEATRICE FOSTER

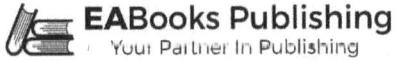

Unlossable Love, (No Matter How Hard You Try)
Copyright @ 2023 John Boyanowski and Beatrice Foster

All rights reserved. No part of this publication may be reproduced or transmitted in any form or by any electronic or mechanical means including photo copying, recording, or any information storage and retrieval system now known or to be invented, without permission in writing from the publisher or the author.

All scriptures from *The Holy Bible*, English Standard Version. ESV® Text Edition: 2016. Copyright © 2001 by Crossway Bibles, a publishing ministry of Good News Publishers.

ISBN: 978-1-955309-63-9
LCCN: 9781955309639

Cover design: Robin Black
Cover photos: Love/Crown of Thorns and Dove/Tomb, iStockphoto/artplus; Jesus Hug, iStockphoto/Motortion

Published by EA Books Publishing, a division of
Living Parables of Central Florida, Inc. a 501c3
EABooksPublishing.com

DEDICATION

This book is dedicated to God, from whom all blessings flow. Because of Him using Beatrice and myself to develop the concept of this book, all praise should be given to Him. From Him, we know and experience *Unlossable Love* in its purest and most excellent way.

Next, to Beatrice Foster: If it weren't for you discovering and developing the phrase *Unlossable Love* and then sharing it, this book would not be possible. Thank you for sharing this with me and for living it out with those in your care and life.

I would also like to thank several individuals who shared their experiences from their past to assist me in showing the power of *Unlossable Love* in their lives. Their stories are examples of how love transforms a life. Dawn Folsom, Justin Davis, and Katelyn Albert thank you for your stories and for being willing to help others with your experiences.

Finally, to my wife Marsha: You have always shown and continue to show this *Unlossable Love* to me throughout the years.

PREFACE

It happened on a Tuesday evening at the beginning of 2022 . . . I was leading a Foster Parent Support Group training in a small town in Indiana. This support group was small in attendance, yet it had more of an impact on me than I ever expected. After all, I was the group's instructor this evening and was to be educating those in attendance about various aspects of foster parenting.

During one of the discussion segments, a young couple, Beatrice and Kenneth Foster were sharing a recent incident involving one of their foster children. As I listened to their story and how they handled the issue, Beatrice made a statement that *instantly* and *completely* captivated me. Beatrice had used the phrase *"Unlossable Love."* God thrust this phrase into my heart, and I had to abruptly interrupt Beatrice to repeat the phrase. (I wanted to make sure I had heard it right.) Beatrice again stated the phrase: I had goose bumps all over my body! Yes, I know it sounds silly; however, this is how God works with me from time to time. (I will go into this in great detail in later chapters.)

Since that time, I have become obsessed with the phrase: I have written an article about it, made a sermon series, and now I am writing this book. (I asked Beatrice for permission to use the phrase and her story.) As you read this book, it is my prayer that God will use it to give you hope and encouragement as you are able to find your value and worth in God and yourself. It is also my hope (as well as Beatrice's) that this will help you to see how great the love of the Father has towards us and that this love, especially from God's point of view, is that *Unlossable Love* that we search for all of our lives. This love can be mirrored in us and through us as we develop the understanding of what *Unlossable Love* is exactly, how to develop it, and how to share it with those we love.

It should be noted that *Unlossable Love* is written from the viewpoint of God's love toward us. This is because this is the very nature of God:

> *Beloved, let us love one another, for love is from God, and whoever loves has been born of God and knows God. Anyone who does not love does not know God, because God is love. In this the love of God was made manifest among us, that God sent his only Son into the world, so that we might live through him. In this is love, not that we have loved God but that he loved us and sent his Son to be the propitiation for our sins. Beloved, if God so loved us, we also ought to love one another. No one has ever seen God; if we love one another, God abides in us and his love is perfected in us.*
>
> *By this we know that we abide in him and he in us, because he has given us of his Spirit. And we have seen and testified that the Father has sent his Son to be the Savior of the world. Whoever confesses that Jesus is the Son of God, God abides in him, and he in God. So we have come to know and to believe the love that God has for us. God is love, and whoever abides in love abides in God, and God abides in him. By this is love perfected with us, so that we may have confidence for the day of judgment, because as he is so also are we in this world. There is no fear in love, but perfect love casts out fear. For fear has to do with punishment, and whoever fears has not been perfected in love. (1 John 4:7–18)*

It is easy for God to possess this form of love because He is love and it is His very nature. Mankind, on the other hand, their nature often contradicts God's nature by their actions and attitudes due to effects of sin on our lives. Does this mean that we have no hope of developing this *Unlossable Love*? Absolutely not! It simply means that we have a great deal of work ahead of us to develop, utilize and *maintain* the *Unlossable Love* we seek to receive and offer to others. Once you understand and experience this type of love, I believe it will be life-changing in many ways (which I will elaborate on in the book). May God richly bless you with His *Unlossable Love* and may He encourage you to teach this love to others.

TABLE OF CONTENTS

How Unlossable Love Came to Be—Beatrice's Story 1
    What Exactly Is Unlossable Love? 8
    What Can Unlossable Love Do for Us? 12
    How Does Unlossable Love Compare to Agape
        (Unconditional) Love? 21
God: The Author of Unlossable Love 27
Man's Search for Love or What One Believes is Love 31
What God's Unlossable Love Means to Us. 39
Is Mankind Capable of Unlossable Love? 46
Unlossable Love and Tainted Pasts 58
Unlossable Love Towards Other 65
Unlossable Love Towards Ourselves 72
Biblical Examples of God's Unlossable Love 79
Developing Our Accessibility to Unlossable Love 86
Cause and Effect of Unlossable Love 95
Overcoming Attitudes Against Unlossable Love 102
Loving the Unlovable 110
Not Faking It till You Make It; Actually Loving the Person(s) 122
Personal, Spiritual, and Mental/Emotional Impacts of Unlossable Love . . 129
When a Person Tries to Run from Unlossable Love 140
When Our Source of Unlossable Love Dies—The Impact 146
Carrying On with Unlossable Love 158
Bonus Feature—Stories from Lives that Experienced Unlossable Love
Dawn's Story 167
Justin's Story 174
Katelyn's Story 183
Final Words 187

HOW *UNLOSSABLE LOVE* CAME TO BE—BEATRICE'S STORY

I shared *briefly* in the preface how I came upon *Unlossable Love* through Beatrice during a Foster Parent Support Group, which I was leading. As I prepared to develop this book, I asked Beatrice to share her account with me of how the phrase *Unlossable Love* came into existence. From the first time I heard Beatrice explain the story, I knew this was something *she* needed to share with the world. Beatrice didn't know at the time just how important this concept would become to me and many others. I never realized just how captivating *Unlossable Love* is personally; it has literally changed my pastoral ministry in profound ways which I will explain later in this book. I will focus on Beatrice's story and use her own words.

> "The term Unlossable Love was created in foster care training, in response to a question asked by the leader. I don't remember the question, but I sat trying to make a word for what I was trying to express. A love that cannot be lost.
>
> To explain the term at its simplest (how I explain it to my children): "No matter if you make good choices or bad choices, Mama will always love you." I want my children to know that my love is not contingent on their decisions. They cannot earn my love, nor can they lose my love, my love is a constant."—Beatrice

When I first read this, I both smiled and teared up because of the beauty behind this; first because of the beauty of the heart of Beatrice and her husband Kenneth towards the children they serve in the foster care system and then because I picture this exact grace which God the Father gives each of us who call upon His Name. Think for a moment about this . . . think about a time when you might have "failed" God and thought to yourself, "God, I'm such an idiot for doing this . . . " and you feel that your failure is too great for God to have the ability to forgive or the desire to forgive you. Maybe there is something that you are experiencing presently that you feel is making you think that God loves you less or not as much . . . my question is "Is that God causing you to feel this way or is it yourself? And if not either of these, is it the Church Proper (those churches which are legalistic and shame you rather than heal you) that is producing this? Or is it the way you were raised, and you believe you can't live up to the expectations that others (or yourself) have of you?" As you can see, there are *many* different factors that can influence our self-image/esteem.

"No matter if you make good choices or bad choices, Mama will always love you. I want my children to know that my love is not contingent on their decisions. They cannot earn my love, nor can they lose my love, my love is a constant." This is an important statement to ponder and learn to adopt into our relationship with not only God but with EVERY relationship we engage in. If we investigate love, we discover that love isn't something we turn on or off, and it's not something we can control. Instead, love should control each of us!

Beatrice's statement to her foster/biological children brings comfort and grace to the recipient of this mercy. As I look at this through our Heavenly Father's eyes and make this personal, I hear him echoing this into my heart from the moment of my conception until the present day. Just like God, Beatrice knows that her children will make mistakes and poor choices and through those times, these children will need the *Unlossable Love* that a parent has towards their children to reassure them not only are they loved unconditionally and unendingly; they continue to have value in the relationship that they share with the parent(s).

In order for us to get a clear understanding of what love truly is, we have to have a definition:

¹**love** \'ləv\ *noun*

[Middle English, from Old English *lufu;* akin to Old High German *luba* love, Old English *lēof* dear, Latin *lubēre, libēre* to please]

(before 12th century)

    1 a (1) : strong affection for another arising out of kinship or personal ties <maternal *love* for a child>

    (2) : attraction based on sexual desire : affection and tenderness felt by lovers

    (3) : affection based on admiration, benevolence, or common interests <love for his old schoolmates>

    b : an assurance of love <give her my *love*>

    2 : warm attachment, enthusiasm, or devotion <*love* of the sea>

    3 a : the object of attachment, devotion, or admiration <baseball was his first *love*>

        3 b (1) : a beloved person : DARLING—often used as a term of endearment

        (2) *British*—used as an informal term of address

    4 a : unselfish loyal and benevolent concern for the good of another: as

        (1) : the fatherly concern of God for humankind

        (2) : brotherly concern for others

    b : a person's adoration of God

    5 : a god or personification of love

    6 : an amorous episode : LOVE AFFAIR

    7 : the sexual embrace : COPULATION

8 : a score of zero (as in tennis)

9 : *capitalized, Christian Science* : GOD[1]

As you can see, there are many definitions and explanations of what love is. The entire list of definitions was shared to point out that we can have different types of love for different types of people and express them in a variety of ways.

For this moment, I want to focus on the first definition, which indicates a strong affection for another arising out of kinship or personal ties. In the case of Beatrice, her love towards her children (both biological and foster children; and I would dare add to her husband, Kenneth) is based on this definition and is expressed through her *Unlossable Love* towards them. She is connected to Kenneth through marriage and has chosen to love him because of the connection that they have developed and cultivated throughout the years.

This same love is for their children who now experience this type of love. When foster children entered the picture; they too were invited to experience this love from Beatrice and Kenneth. Please understand that this was a vastly different experience for these foster children who come from dysfunctional families, broken relationships, and various traumas. To these children, love is an overused word that holds no value: those who were supposed to love them have abused this and have left them broken. To these, love is but a unicorn: a myth that is nice to believe in and yet is unattainable.

When a person (any person) has a trust issue with love and the REAL definition of love (defined by God *and* including Webster's definition), it is common for these to have strong doubts about the reality that they can experience such a love. You may find resistance to

---

1   "Love." Merriam-Webster.com Dictionary, Merriam-Webster, https://www.merriam-webster.com/dictionary/compassion. Accessed 20 Jul. 2023.

accepting this love (or any form of love); even though they are starving for this. They resist love because of the pain which the broken promise that love is forever, they might have been manipulated by those who claim to love them, or they might have witnessed the abuse of love in their parent(s)'s life or someone close to them. This, along with the possibility of having low/no self-esteem, a sense of value or even living with guilt because of poor choices/mistakes, create a great barrier that some might use to protect their hearts/souls or to self-punish their choices.

I can and do identify with this because I had a "dysfunctional" family (which I perceived at the time). In our family, alcohol played a devastating role in how I viewed love and how to obtain love. I saw firsthand how this substance caused division, anger, broken trust and promises, and a lack of self-esteem. I never felt valued because I thought it was the alcohol that made my father like me; if he couldn't engage with me except under the influence, I didn't want the interaction with him.

This followed me into adulthood when people I dated would try to engage with me and express love in whatever ways they did: If they were under the influence of substances, I wanted no part of the engagement because I felt that they were only engaging with me in this fashion because of the substances and not because my value to them when they were sober.

My thoughts at that time were, "Why do they have to drink/use substances to be with me? Am I that unlovable that they need to be drunk/stoned to love me?"

I never said it was rational thinking, yet this is what many may think when such events take place. I would refuse to engage with the individual because if they couldn't stay sober while with me, I wanted no part of their activities while they were under the influence.

I had thought that real love was impossible for me, to the point of forsaking love together. I vowed to never allow love into my life because when real love is removed, it is the greatest pain one can experience.

I refused to accept and give love for a time. Someone would confess their love, and I would simply ignore their statements or even tell them to refrain from such comments.

The hurt and pain of the removal of love that drove me to this point had corrupted my soul and mind to force me to believe I am unworthy of real love. After all, I've been hurt by the best of them (those who are supposed to love you with the *Unlossable Love* which I now write about). I refused love from family, friends, and even God Himself! I shortly began to notice a *physical* change: I was experiencing increased chest pains, being tired easily, fast pulse rate—at the age of 17 years old! I didn't understand what was going on with me or my body.

Then God somehow connected with me . . . I would like to say how He did it, but I can't say for certain just how He did it. For some reason, I was reading my Bible when these verses came to me at just the right time:

> *"So we have come to know and to believe the love that God has for us. God is love, and whoever abides in love abides in God, and God abides in him. By this is love perfected with us, so that we may have confidence for the day of judgment, because as he is so also are we in this world. There is no fear in love, but perfect love casts out fear. For fear has to do with punishment, and whoever fears has not been perfected in love." (1 John 4:15–18)*

I must have read these verses a million times (I know that it was only literally several hundred times, but I continue to read and share these verses with all I can)—just trying to understand and absorb the meanings and grace which comes with it. Verse 18 of 1 John captivated me to the point that this is now my life verse. Please allow me to break it down into various parts of the understanding which God graced me with.

There is no fear in love . . .—Because of past bad experiences, I feared love, as shared earlier. I wanted to argue and prove God a fool because of these experiences, and I could find *plenty* of others who would agree with me on this point. I couldn't believe such a love could ever exist; especially for me. Yes, I dreamed of such love and fantasized that maybe one day I could possibly experience it.

Due to my past, I knew I was only lying to myself. God haunted my thoughts and dreams directly after the first time of reading this verse. My thoughts slowly turned from "No way in hell . . ." to, "What if . . .?" I tried to convince myself of the *probability* of such love as I continued to read...

. . . But perfect love casts out fear.—Perfect love? I thought I had experienced this a thousand times over. Call it immaturity, inexperience, being naïve, or whatever, I knew what love was. As I continued to reread this part of the verse, the Holy Spirit began to teach me that all the various forms of love had a great deal of imperfections: They caused pain, abandonment, had stipulations attached to it (both from others and my own stipulations), had produced fear of its loss from my life, produced manipulations in various forms, and a host of other effects. Even when it didn't affect me directly, I had witnessed this in many different lives, including my parents' lives. I heard that "There's no such thing as a 'perfect' love," and at the same time, we hear in fairy tales that such love is possible for everyone. So, what is *perfect love*? Here is how I view it today:

- *Agape* (unconditional)—There aren't any expectations attached to it: this prevents any form of manipulation from taking place.
- *Unlossable*—Nothing we do or say can erode it or destroy it, it stays consistent with or even increases throughout time.
- *It is a gift*—it can't be bought, earned, or anything except offered freely by the giver of this love.
- *The gift is accepted and utilized*—The gift must be accepted in order for it to be a gift. And the appreciation of the gift is to use

the gift as it is intended to be used. To accept the gift and not use it is to defer the blessing it was intended to be. It becomes a "collectible" more than a blessing. Blessings are active and engaging; most collectibles are not.

- *There is no fear*—We understand that utilizing this gift will produce what it is intended to do. It is *evidence-based*, meaning that when utilized properly, the same result will take place *each and every time*. A perfect love can't be broken, ended, or forfeited by either party—the giver or the receiver. Once love is established, especially by God, it is for eternity.

Sounds like a dream, but God makes it a reality because He is that Love. Regardless of what we do in this life; even if we *never* accept God's love for our own doesn't change the love He has for us. If we choose a path that leads to Hell, God *continues to love us*. (One might ask, "If He loves us so, why would He send someone to Hell?" If we choose to be separated from Him and His love and remain that way through our time of death, then we have chosen to remain apart from Him in eternity. It is *our desire* to be estranged from God. He *always* has and *always* will love us with *Unlossable Love*, enough to give us what our heart desires. The natural consequence for such desires follows us even into death.) God loves us, period. Nothing—death, Hell, or anything else—can and will separate us from this love. This leads us to our next chapter. . . .

What Exactly Is *Unlossable Love*?

Before we dive into what *Unlossable Love* exactly is, allow me to remind you what Beatrice's definition is:

To explain the term at its simplest (how I explain it to my children): "No matter if you make good choices or bad choices,

How Unlossable Love Came to Be—Beatrice's Story

Mama will always love you." I want my children to know that my love is not contingent on their decisions. They cannot earn my love, nor can they lose my love, my love is a constant."—Beatrice

Now we can build on this and make it a deeper understanding of what I believe is the heart of the definition. *Unlossable Love* is just that—a love that one can never shake off or lose. Ponder on this for a second or two . . . can you begin to comprehend such love?

Many, if not all of us, can relate to a time or two (for some, even more) when we believed we had a love and for some reason or another, that love was forsaken. A breakup, someone moving away from you and you lost contact with one another, death, divorce, addictions that caused the relationship to end, a change of heart, domestic violence, abuse of all sorts, mental illness (as in dementia, Alzheimer's disease, bipolar and other . . .), traumas, low/no self-esteem, and more can and does contribute to the death/loss of a loving relationship. When this occurs, the devastation that it leaves behind in a soul can and often does cause "endless" effects on a person at *any* age (the reason for the quotation marks with "endless" will be explained later in this chapter). The person feels abandoned, rejected, worthless, undesirable, and nonexistent. This feeling changes the reality of the person to feel that love, *real love*, is never meant for them.

This is where I will draw from my experiences in working with the foster care system to explain the thoughts of one's self-perception and how easy it is for a person to believe in such a distorted reality. Children are placed in the foster care system for a variety of reasons. A common perception is that most of the foster children's parents are addicts of some substance or that the parents are abusing the children in extreme measures. These do make up the majority of the reasons for removal, but the reasons go even deeper, and the causes are deeper still.

The children are taken from the parents; the very ones who are supposed to care/love/protect them from being harmed and these are the very people causing the pain! (In defense of the parents, they themselves most likely are victims as well and know no better because of generational patterns of abuse and neglect. They respond by what they have experienced and have no real understanding of what a healthy family relationship is like.) The children are removed from the parents and are brought, in most instances, to complete strangers in what are strange places to the children and are exposed to a completely different family system and are told to adapt to this new environment. Just in this short explanation, the children has experienced several different traumas. At this point, the trauma experienced has stagnated the children and has created confusion, helplessness, and hopelessness, and they begin to question *everything* about their lives.

It doesn't stop there . . . nor does the carnage from the event. Some might begin to ask if *they* themselves were the cause of the removal: "If I was a better kid, maybe we never would have been taken from Mom and Dad." "If I would listen better maybe mom/dad wouldn't need to drink/use drugs." "If I didn't show my bruises to someone, we would still be together."

These are all but a few thoughts that run through the minds of the foster children. Please understand that at the same time, the parents of these beloved children *also* struggle with the loss of love and experience similar devastation to which their children fall victim. The single parent has dysfunctional relationships and because of lack of/no love or self-esteem, allows the dysfunction to occur because no matter how bad they are treated, they "at least have someone who says they love them." (Although this is an unhealthy relationship, they view it as being better than having no relationship at all.)

As stated earlier, the parents might have experienced trauma in the past that they haven't dealt with and struggled with the brokenness of their own. In their eyes, *Unlossable Love* has never existed because they can't fathom that real love possibly existed in their lives. One might use the term "love," however, the understanding of love escapes them.

To add to what Beatrice expresses of *Unlossable Love*, this is a love that is established with no expiration dates, no "best used by" dates, or conditions attached to them. *Unlossable Love* is not watered down when things go wrong. It is not a love that decreases but *increases* with every breath; especially when trials and tribulations come (which calls for an increase of love and compassion). This love doesn't overlook or forsake what wrongs are done; *Unlossable Love* walks side by side with the individual until the full restoration has taken place. This love doesn't hesitate to step in and take action to protect the individual from falling deeper into their poor decisions and lifestyle choices. As described in 1 Corinthians:

> *If I speak in the tongues of men and of angels, but have not love, I am a noisy gong or a clanging cymbal. And if I have prophetic powers, and understand all mysteries and all knowledge, and if I have all faith, so as to remove mountains, but have not love, I am nothing. If I give away all I have, and if I deliver up my body to be burned, but have not love, I gain nothing.*
>
> *Love is patient and kind; love does not envy or boast; it is not arrogant or rude. It does not insist on its own way; it is not irritable or resentful; it does not rejoice at wrongdoing, but rejoices with the truth. Love bears all things, believes all things, hopes all things, endures all things.*
>
> *Love never ends. (1 Corinthians 13:1–8)*

I can picture this as God's explanation of *Unlossable Love*. When you look at the explanation of what love is, you can behold a beautiful picture of what is possible in love and because of love. Man has placed various limits and conditions on love, using love as a weapon or a controlling device to capture hopeful prey in its grasp. This passage shows just the opposite: the control is squarely placed upon not the receiver of the love, but on the one sharing the love.

At no point does the writer of 1 Corinthians state that these are the requirements one should expect. The apostle Paul, the writer, gives the readers the definition and characteristics of love, and with it, the expectation that true love is a receptacle between all parties involved. It is to be understood that with this form of love, and the importance of equal commitment from all, will make this love an *Unlossable Love*. Why? Because love holds no records of wrong. Love bears all things. Love believes in all things. Love hopes for all things. Love endures all things. Love *never* ends. Sounds like *Unlossable Love to me*.

What Can *Unlossable Love* Do for Us?

In the last chapter, we discussed the definition of what *Unlossable Love* might be considered through the eyes of God. Now, let's look at what exactly it is when it is practiced and applied to an individual's life. Again, we will engage with Beatrice's story; this time involving an individual which whom she had been friends (names were changed to not break any confidentiality):

> The first time I witnessed this love in action, in an earthly manner, was with a friend of mine, Meredith. We attended the same church at the time, and both of us were raised in the church. Her father was the head pastor, and my father was an elder. I was asked to give my testimony at a lady's retreat.
>
> I didn't go into details, but I explained that I was raised in the church, left for 10 years, and had come back. I gave the invitation that if anyone wanted to hear the details of why I had left, they could speak to me one on one.
>
> Meredith approached me later and asked if we could meet for coffee; we set up our coffee date for the following Thursday. As we sat having coffee, Meredith started telling me all the "bad"

things she was secretly involved in, things that the church would look down upon her for.

I sat and listened and started sharing my story. I could match almost everything she said. Meredith was raised in a church, full of head knowledge of Christ, but she was taught as a child that her worth/love was contingent on her performance. The result of that teaching was a young woman contemplating suicide because she sought love/acceptance and couldn't find it. She asked if I would mentor her; she needed a big sister.

We parted ways that evening with the plan to re-meet Sunday morning. I went home and prayed for her; my heart was so heavy for her. We met on Sunday, as planned. I explained to her that I would be happy to mentor her. My exact words were "You have two paths ahead of you, one you can choose God and choose to follow what He says, or you can choose the world. No matter your decision, I will mentor you."

I didn't know how much that conversation meant to her until years later. As our relationship grew, I invited her into my home for meals and to spend time with my family. We didn't ask where she had been, or what choices she was making; we just accepted her and treated her as one of our family. She eventually decided to follow God.

A year later she was looking for a home. She could live with her parents, but they made it clear that her standing with them was contingent on her life choices. If she couldn't meet their standards, she would find her things in the driveway. Kenneth and I offered her a home with us, and she lived with us until God called her to other adventures. We are still in contact with her daily. She serves God faithfully and loves others in her community, her calling is to accept and love abused and hard people, people of trauma. I am happy to say that her parents and she have rectified the relationship, it's not perfect, but what in this life really is?"

The very first aspect of *Unlossable Love* is to develop the mindset of commitment: committing to be there for the long hall. Beatrice understood how important committing to someone truly transforms a life.

Because of various life experiences, along with her and her husband, Kenneth, being foster parents, Beatrice has worked with individuals whose lives were devastated and put asunder. The various traumas, broken relationships, and abandonments of various manners have sucked the souls out of these cherished people. Because of this, these cherished people were traumatized by their experiences. Their pain and brokenness had been so destructive that they consciously/subconsciously disabled their ability to love and accept love. Their ability to feel any trust from anyone was turned off in order to save themselves from ever experiencing this level of rejection or suffering.

Regaining a level of trust, even the smallest level, might take a great deal of time and effort on our part. Especially in the various cases in which I had been involved with foster children, juvenile delinquents, and others, these have done a number of negative actions to avoid anyone attempting to become close with them. It is their belief, in many cases, that if they act negatively, they will chase away those trying to love them; thus, they will give up on them and leave them alone. This is a defensive move to keep people from trying to break their hearts. Beatrice shares an example:

> Kenneth and I are foster parents. Primarily we have been placed with smaller children, but one night in 2019, we were placed with a 10-year-old boy named Troy. Troy was a hard kid; he lived a life of defeat and chaos.

Troy couldn't understand how he was part of our family, because we weren't blood. He couldn't understand the love I was offering him. I told him what I tell all my kids, "No matter what you choose to do, I will always love you."

Troy wanted to believe and accept my love, but he couldn't. He eventually started hurting me emotionally, to the point I wanted death, instead of the morning, to come. Kenneth had to interfere, and we had to have Troy move to another home.

I refused to let him go to another foster home. Part of his trauma was that whenever his father and his father's girlfriends would break up, his father would tell Troy that it was his fault. That is a lot to put on the shoulders of a child. I knew that if Troy had to move from my home because of his behavior, he would take the blame and relive the trauma of his youth.

So instead, we started shaking his family tree and praying. Thank you, Lord, we eventually found a distant cousin who was willing and able to welcome Troy into his home. Troy moved on with a new lease on life; he was wanted and desired by his own family, and he was still loved by us.

I heard from Troy from time to time, and one day I received a letter from him. In his letter, he asked me how I could love him despite how he treated me. Why had I loved him even when he hurt me? I wrote him back and explained that it was only because of Jesus and Jesus' love for me that I was able to extend that love to him. Troy is doing ok now. He is still struggling with his trauma and will be for a while.

Troy is like millions of others who experience various forms of abuse, trauma, and neglect from a variety of life experiences—bullying, addictions, poor choices which isolated himself from others, abandonment, and so on. These experiences will cause our hearts to harden quicker than lightning and more solidly than the Rock of Gibraltar.

And like in Troy's case, it will take great patience and time to even begin to soften the hearts in the smallest of ways. In some cases, the individual has control of their decisions; while in other cases, their ability to choose is robbed from them by others. However, if we are willing to invest time and effort into these broken souls, God can and will restore and heal the person who desires to be healed.

The next step in *Unlossable Love* is compassion: to try and understand who they are, what they came from, who they want to be, and being nonjudgmental at the same time.

By doing this step, we are able to assess how ready the individual is to accept the *Unlossable Love* that we are trying to establish; as well as to be able to discover the various ways to apply this love to the individual. As we understand the circumstances that have brought them to this point, it assists us to be less judgmental.

Let's face it, it's human nature to be judgmental, and even the best of us have predetermined biases and judgments against various actions, beliefs, and experiences, which cause us to be prejudiced in some way. These prejudices are not limited to race/color but can be political, theological, gender orientated, criminal activities (such as rapists, murderers, domestic violence, etc.), and more. These thoughts and beliefs can destroy compassion—especially when it involves us, someone that we love, for those who have been victimized by such actions.

What exactly is compassion? The world will give you many variations of what compassion is, but we will use the following definitions:

COMPASSION: Quality of showing kindness or favor, of being gracious, or of having pity or mercy. In the Bible, God is described as a compassionate father to those who revere him (Ps. 103:13). Jesus Christ exemplified God's compassion in his preaching and healing (Mt. 9:36; 14:14), in his concern for the lostness of humanity (Lk. 19:41), and finally in his sacrifice on the cross (Rom. 5:8). The church is to demonstrate compassion as one facet of the love Jesus commanded (Mt. 5:4–7; Jn. 13:34; Jas. 2:8–18; 1 Jn. 3:18). In scriptural usage, compassion is always both a feeling and the appropriate action based on that feeling.[2]

> **com•pas•sion** \kəm-ˈpa-shən\ *noun*
>
> [Middle English, from Middle French or Late Latin; Middle French, from Late Latin *compassion-, compassio,* from *compati* to sympathize, from Latin *com-* + *pati* to bear, suffer — more at PATIENT]
>
> (14th century)
>
> : sympathetic consciousness of other's distress together with a desire to alleviate it[3]

Compassion, for all of us and not just someone else, is a key element for *Unlossable Love*. It is a foundational platform that solidifies the ability for the application of love/healing to take place. Like foster parents, there are many people with similar hearts and minds in which compassion is their life essence. And these are not just those with a religion or faith-based; these are individuals who see injustices and trauma in others and believe they are gifted with compassion and desire to bring some sort of peace and value to those who may never have had such dignity presented to them.

Next, we want to present questions. Why is this the next step? Simply put, we must know how to ask the right questions to be able to give the right assistance at the right time. Jesus is known to have been a man who would ask questions:

---

[2] Elwell, W. A., & Comfort, P. W., *Tyndale Bible Dictionary,* (Carol Stream, Ill.: Tyndale House Publishers, 2008), 306.
[3] "Compassion." Merriam-Webster.com Dictionary, Merriam-Webster, https://www.merriam-webster.com/dictionary/compassion. Accessed 20 Jul. 2023.

> *"Or which one of you, if his son asks him for bread, will give him a stone? Or if he asks for a fish, will give him a serpent?"(Matthew 7:9–10)*
>
> *"Why do you ask me about what is good?"(Matthew 19:17)*
>
> *"When Jesus saw him lying there and knew that he had already been there a long time, he said to him, "Do you want to be healed?" (John 5:6)*

Asking questions will allow us to be able to see the heart of the individual with whom we are trying to connect. We do not want to presume that we know exactly what they're thinking and feeling and then discover that we have done more harm because we haven't listened to what their hearts were saying. We want to have clarification as to what is going on in their life, where they feel that they need assistance or help, and then try to achieve the goals that they have set for themselves.

It is at that point that we try to teach about *Unlossable Love* and how it can be theirs, because we have already established the other foundations, trust, and demonstrated active and reflective listening. When a person feels heard, they often feel validated as a person because somebody has listened to them, sometimes for the very first time in their life.

This next statement may sound a bit crazy, however, it is a very important statement that will assist you to be prepared: Expect battles.

As we all know, change is difficult at times. We like to have more consistency than inconsistency because it makes us feel more comfortable and we know what to expect. When regular people have sudden changes in routines, they sometimes get flustered and will become unfocused. Now, consider someone who was just ripped from their home, school, friends, faith systems, and so on and then are thrust into foster care. The very ones who are charged to care for them sometimes become the very perpetrators of the traumas they face. Those who were supposed to give the *Unlossable Love* are the same ones who have deemed them "unworthy", "unlovable", and "will never amount to anything."

Now, these same children who are thrust into a stranger's home and family, into a different culture with conflicting belief systems from their own, now going to a strange school, with strange people who look at them as different (and if they are found out to be "foster kids," they are teased and tormented), and there is no set time for possible reunification with family members. These individuals will cause a battle because they have no control over their situations and what little control they had in their lives has been stolen by "the system." *They will battle!* It might not be at first; but rest assured, a battle is coming. If we are not prepared for it, *we* might be the ones who lose control, along with the children. Adults experience this too.

People fight because they are scared. They fight because they want some form of control, any form of control over their life. Some people have had little to no control at all because others have dominated their lives, victimized them, and have left them emotionally dead. They may even fight themselves: They battled the demons that they have within themselves that are disguised as mental illness, depression, anxieties, and worries, and this should also be added, spiritual battles.

People will fight themselves because of past environmental and social biases, which tried to dominate their way of thought and belief. If a person is honest with themselves, they will understand that these battles are the most severe because they can be well hidden behind the mask that most people will place on their face: a smile.

There are many who tried to present themselves as having no cares in the world; when they are internally battling legions of fears and anxieties that have rooted themselves into their very souls. For many, these battles are very real, very intense, and as in all battles, are completely devastating. Although nobody enjoys going to battle; these battles are necessary because they will challenge the way we think and feel about ourselves and our relationships. These battles should be able to expose weaknesses in our relationships and our thoughts about these same relationships that we strive to have in our lives. When these weaknesses are exposed, and if these are the relationships, we wish to nurture with *Unlossable Love*, we can now have a foundation of where we need to start the repairs. At the same time, exposure to weaknesses can produce relationships that could become toxic and deadly emotionally.

It should be noted here that even as we expose these forms of relationships, as God directs us to, we should be using this information to protect our hearts and at the same time, allow ourselves to be vulnerable enough to form these new relationships. *Unlossable Love* is possible only when we allow ourselves the ability to develop that love with ourselves from God, and then transfer it to those individuals who need it the most. These individuals may have been fighting against love because of the multiple times their hearts have been broken and manipulated, as well as being traumatized, to the point where they never want to hurt again.

These experiences make it hard to trust in others and there will be strong adversities that they will use to guard their hearts against any more onslaughts of trauma. We try to teach and educate these individuals how to trust not only in others but also believe in themselves, that they are worthy of receiving love that is long-lasting and asks nothing in return. For some, it may be an easy transition because they are starving for the *Unlossable Love* being offered. Others will try to fight with every breath within their being against this love because of the depths of the trauma they have experienced. It is a very understandable response to what is happening in their lives. And still, others haven't a clue as to the need for such a love in their lives because they have been taught and trained that love comes and goes like the tides of the ocean.

Now that we have a better understanding of what *Unlossable Love* is, how does this compare to God's Agape Love (unconditional love)?

How Does *Unlossable Love* Compare to Agape (Unconditional) Love?

Agape

    agape (ah-gah′pay), the principal Greek word used for 'love' in the NT. Of the three words for love in the Hellenistic world, it was the least common. The other two words were *eros*, which meant sexual love, and *philos*, which meant friendship, although their meanings could vary according to the context in which they appeared. Agape, because it was used so seldom and was so unspecific in meaning, could be used in the NT to designate the unmerited love God shows to humankind in sending his son as suffering redeemer. When used of human love, it means selfless and self-giving love[4]

Using Beatrice's explanation of *Unlossable Love*:

> *"To explain the term at its simplest (how I explain it to my children): "No matter if you make good choices or bad choices, Mama will always love you." I want my children to know that my love is not contingent on their decisions. They cannot earn my love, nor can they lose my love, my love is a constant."*—Beatrice

To the average person, there are consistencies between both agape love and *Unlossable Love* that could lead one to believe that they are the same. However, there are two distinctions that make these two terms different: Agape love is unconditional and unmerited grace that

---

4 Achtemeier, P. J., *Harper's Bible Dictionary*, (San Francisco: Harper & Row, 1985), 14.

is given to all people. If they should accept this agape love, it can create the greatest miracle in their lives.

Unlossable Love, much like God's agape love, is an unconditional love that the person receives even if they choose not to accept it. God never forces His will on anyone and allows the individual to accept or decline this gift. God never removes His offer from mankind, and when the individual is ready to accept it, that is when the agape love can transform life as we know it.

Unlossable Love, however, although it remains constant much like agape love, causes the individual giving this love to an individual to be *actively engaged* with the individual in their struggles to learn and understand exactly what love is and is not. It must be noted here that *Unlossable Love* isn't being forced upon anyone; the individual is becoming combative with the one dispersing the love. The individual chooses to reject all forms of love and trust because of the fear of being hurt once again and, if the individual was traumatized badly enough, the individual will do everything in their power to destroy that love before it destroys them.

It seems crazy, but the reality is we have many people who have been traumatized so much by those who are expected to protect their best interest are the actual victimizers which destroyed their love and trust. This trauma can be overcome, but it will take both God's agape love and His/our *Unlossable Love* to bring full restoration into the individual's life.

It should be noted here that God is the author and creator of *Unlossable Love* through His agape love. This type of love is misunderstood because of man's prerequisites that they place on love in the various definitions thereof. *Love* is a term which man uses the most and is the most misused term in all the languages of the earth. Love seems to have lost its importance because we use that term for everything, and we assume that love has only one meaning. We say that we love our spouse, and we love cheeseburgers. We say we love the Boston Red Sox (my favorite baseball team!), and at the same time, we love our parents. We love our pets, and we love our movies. As you can see by these examples, we are talking about various forms of love and various intensities of the way we love.

Obviously, we will admit that we love our spouse far greater than a cheeseburger (and if you don't, please seek professional help, LOL). As much as I love the Boston Red Sox, my love for my parents far outweighs my passion for my baseball team. The love we have for our pets far outweighs the love that we have for any movie; would you give up your pet to be able to go see a movie? Obviously not! Because the term love has been used so flippantly, it has lost its impact in all the various meanings that it represents and become meaningless.

In the same way that agape love incorporates *Unlossable Love*, the same can be said as you reverse the two. *Unlossable Love* must have its foundation built upon God's agape love in order for it to stand. Without the agape foundation, this love could be misinterpreted by the receiver of this love. As Beatrice and Kenneth lived out the example of *Unlossable Love* for their children, foster children, and each other, it had to be understood by all that the love that they have for each other is not based upon what each other can do for one another (causing them to think that they can earn this love), but that this love continually exists because of God's love for us and His example towards us through His agape love.

In an earlier chapter, we have been able to establish that God is love. He has existed from all eternity to all eternity. God has placed within every one of us that same ability to have that same type of love not only by God and from God, but to also have it for one another, should we so choose. The difference is man has used and abused this love and continues to do so today. The foster children that Beatrice and Kenneth work with are prime examples of this. And, sadly to say, there are millions more who are silently suffering the same experience. It has been ingrained in individuals that they have to earn their love from others by becoming whatever the others want them to become. This is not love.

With agape love, there are no conditions required. God gives us this love as a gift. Even if we reject this love, God's love remains. I have preached that God's love is so divine and so perfect for us that even if we should end up in hell, God does not stop loving us. You might ask, "If God loves us so, why do we go to hell?" The answer is very simple: God loves us so much that he gives us what we asked for.

If, while we are still alive, we choose to distance ourselves from God all of our lives, and we never ask Him to come into our lives while we still have breath on this earth, it is our choice that kept us separated from Him. Since we have not asked him to come into our lives while we were alive, we will continue our separation from God after we die. God's agape love continues to pursue us and hopes that it will have the ability to transform us should we allow it to. God continually brings people and circumstances into our lives to show the importance of accepting this love before it becomes too late for us. Up until our final breath, God continues to remind us of his love that while we were yet sinners, Christ died for us.

> *"For while we were still weak, at the right time Christ died for the ungodly. For one will scarcely die for a righteous person— though perhaps for a good person one would dare even to die— but God shows his love for us in that while we were still **sinners**, Christ died for us."(Romans 5:6–8)*

God's agape love is demonstrated in these verses. It is this foundation that we attached to *Unlossable Love* to make both even stronger than we can imagine. There are no prerequisites and no expectations as we present both forms of love to the individuals in our lives.

Another way in which agape love and *Unlossable Love* compares is found in First Corinthians 13:

> *"If I speak in the tongues of men and of angels, but have not love, I am a noisy gong or a clanging cymbal. And if I have prophetic powers, and understand all mysteries and all knowledge, and if I have all faith, so as to remove mountains, but have not love, I am nothing. If I give away all I have, and if I deliver up my body to be burned, but have not love, I gain nothing.*
>
> *Love is patient and kind; love does not envy or boast; it is not arrogant or rude. It does not insist on its own way; it is not irritable or resentful; it does not rejoice at wrongdoing, but rejoices with the truth. Love bears all things, believes all things, hopes all things, endures all things.*
>
> *Love never ends." (1 Corinthians 13:1–8)*

When Paul writes to the Corinthian church, he shares about what love is according to God. As you look at the definitions found between verses 4–8, we get the opportunity to see how love ought to be. Many of us in loving relationships may not even have a clue that these verses exist, and yet, these are the core values of what love should be.

Now, try to explain these to individuals who have been traumatized by those who would claim to love them and have let them down repeatedly. The walls go up around their hearts and imprison them in solitary confinement emotionally, and sometimes spiritually, so that they will never feel the effects of a lost love ever again.

These people get used to being in solitude (or so they claim) and consider this to be the cure for what ails them. Then when we attempt to introduce them to the real cure, some attempt to build even stronger walls because of their fear. As we teach individuals these verses found in the Scriptures, we help them to know that God's plan never meant for anyone to be without love, assurance, and value. These traits cultivate and fertilize the seed of love that can be planted in an individual's life. I truly appreciate Paul's statement

Unlossable Love

at the beginning of verse eight: "Love never fails." This is where agape love and *Unlossable Love* unite to form the salvation of the soul and their ability to love.

GOD: THE AUTHOR OF UNLOSSABLE LOVE

It was stated in the last chapter that God is the author of *Unlossable Love* and rightfully so. Although He used Beatrice and Kenneth to plant the seed for this generation, this love has been around since the beginning of creation. We have just finished the comparison between agape love and this love in the former chapter and noted how they compare to one another and how important one is to the other and vice versa.

Man did not create *Unlossable Love*; God has through Himself. We see this lived out in the life of Christ as He engaged the world that one week would praise Him and exalt Him as King, and then in less than a week would despise Him and do unspeakable things to Him. And even in the midst of all of this, Jesus would pray for those who were persecuting Him and ask God to forgive them.

Jesus Himself felt the betrayal of love and was abandoned by those who claimed to love Him endlessly. This did not deter Jesus from love and all of mankind dying for their sins. Jesus, being very much human as well as being very much God, could have taken on man's mindset and place conditions upon those whom He loves. Jesus could have easily said that He was only dying for those who love Him. Thank God that Jesus maintained agape and *Unlossable Love*! This same love continues thousands of years later and will continue throughout all of eternity.

Did God create this love for mankind *only* for when Jesus roamed the earth? Absolutely not! For us to understand when it first began, we must explore the origins of creation. In the book of Genesis, we read the creation story where God had formed the heavens and the earth and all that is within. When God made man, in contrast to all things that were created before him, God made the simple statement that those things were "good." However, when God made mankind, He noted that it was "very good." This goes to show a very important relationship that would take place between God and man.

If one believes that God is all-knowing, all-powerful, in all and through all, then it should be noted that God would know man's condition and his falling away from grace during the Garden experience (Genesis chapter 3). God knew that sin would enter the hearts of men even before man was created and still created them anyway.

Why would he do this? Simply put, because of God's agape and *Unlossable Love* towards us. God became both forms of love because God knew that both forms of love are needed in the redemption of a man's soul. For this reason, Satan tries so desperately to convince individuals of how unlovable they are and how worthless they are in hopes to try to keep them separated from God.

Satan cares nothing for man and completely loathes God and the best way for him to get back at God is to separate God from the creation that he loves most: mankind. If Satan can convince a man that he is worthless to God and to one another, he can control man's heart and manipulate him to do his bidding. Because God is love, He bestows his agape love and *Unlossable Love* on us to reveal to us how precious we are to Him.

When I spoke with Beatrice about her concept of *Unlossable Love*, we both understood that this was a God thing taking place. We both ask ourselves why God would reveal this to us. I know for Beatrice, she needed this to bless and restore her family and those that she and Kenneth would foster.

As I shared at the beginning of the book, this concept and outlook caused me to have goose bumps all over my body! Immediately, I knew that God was revealing to us something amazing that could transform many lives and could restore the brokenness in so many. I believe that God has chosen Beatrice and Kenneth because He knew that they would be not only obedient to the calling, but they would also share this with others, and I am extremely humbled to be one of those individuals.

I also believe that God is using my gifts and talents to be able to work with Beatrice and Kenneth to put down to words their heart and passion on the importance of *Unlossable Love* and it is utilized in today's generation. As we wait upon the Lord to reveal to myself and the Fosters how this message plays out, we are eager and humbled for this opportunity to bring *Unlossable Love* to the masses. We continue to prayerfully listen to what God places on our hearts and to allow God to be the author of this book. Without God, *Unlossable Love* is just a concept. With God, it becomes a reality and an evidence-based practice that will ultimately impact millions of people as it spreads across the land.

I truly believe that the timing for this book is imperative for this generation to know and understand. I believe that God sees the divisions throughout all of mankind: The family unit being eroded away by absentee fathers or nothing more than sperm donors does not take their responsibility of being a father to their children and how the mothers are sometimes forced to work multiple jobs to try to supply for the needs of the family, the weaponization of social media as a tool of the destruction of individual's self-worth, the avoidance of developing and nurturing of the spiritual self (one's connection with God), the selfishness and greed of not only finances but also power, are just a few of the reasons such a book is in need at this present time.

God is trying to turn our focus towards Himself to reveal Himself through the love that He is. Too many times we tend to focus more on the problems that this life brings than the solution that God brings and is Himself. In addition to this, we tend to busy ourselves with things to escape the reality of the emptiness that we feel inside. It is a great deal easier to ignore an issue than it is to face it; especially when it pertains to matters of the heart.

God sees all of this and more. For this reason, God imparts His love to us. There are times when we fail to see our need for a Savior. We believe ourselves to have the ability to handle things on our own and we fool ourselves into this belief. In doing this, we forfeit the possibilities of connecting with God's agape and *Unlossable Love* because our focus is on healing ourselves.

God has equipped, men and women, as evidenced by Beatrice and Kenneth's example, to be the conduits of His love to share these loves with others. God can also equip each of us to not only be recipients of these loves but to also become conduits to disperse these loves to others. For this to take place, we must first experience firsthand these loves and then model these to whom God places on our hearts (which basically means, everybody we encounter). This is a humble privilege and honor granted to us by God the Author of love.

MAN'S SEARCH FOR LOVE OR WHAT ONE BELIEVES IS LOVE

As early as our infancy (possibly even in the womb if we have parents reading to their babies in the womb), we are taught, in various ways, man's concept of love. These expressions of love within the womb come from the mother singing to her child, rubbing her belly to caress her child within the womb, taking proper care of herself—which in turn takes care of the child within—and telling stories to her child.

Once the child is born, the parents can do the same activities and more face-to-face. They feed and care for the child to the best of their abilities. As the child matures, they are told bedtime stories in which the heroes always rush to save the day in the major characters of the story usually live happily ever after. These kinds of things give us all the warm fuzzies, but are these based, especially for today's generations?

All children are beautiful gifts from God. However, man tends to not appreciate the gifts God gives us. Yes, will love and care for the children up until the point when reality sets in, and we must live life. We have various demands to attend to, and our ability to show consistent love and devotion towards the children shortens as each moment passes. Based upon our lot in life, some of us may have to work several jobs in order to make ends meet. Others of us place ourselves in predicaments or situations that we once thought were positive choices that quickly enslaved us to situations far beyond our capabilities to control. Soon, our fantasies become nightmares and we question how we got where we are today.

Because we are not able to get the intense attention of love as we did in the womb, along with the decrease of attention because our level of need changes on a regular basis, man begins to look for love (or what they perceived to be what love is to them). Based upon those influences on the person's life, one can grow into a very mature individual, or one can be stifled in the development of a clear understanding of love. This is where things become as clear as mud: The individual must decipher for themselves their concept of what love is and is not, as well as try various forms of love to see if they fulfill the need they are looking for.

Because I have worked in the mental health field for numerous years, I have seen and experienced the vast scope in which people search for meaning and purpose from love. I have seen the innocence of a person's soul be presented to individuals who they thought would love them back in the way that they search for—only for them to find out that these individuals whom they trusted were perpetrators of their emotional demise and traumatized them.

I have seen individuals who being denied healthy, loving relationships at the beginning of their life and struggle far into their adulthood to have the ability to develop healthy relationships with others. At the same time, I have also witnessed individuals who had overcome their traumas and became the very individuals that their innocent hearts searched for in their youth/adulthood. These individuals understood what it was like to be unlovable, had other individuals mentor them in discovering the love that they sought, and then trained themselves to become conduits of that love for others. These individuals are a very special group of people who can transform the world around them because they were once in the shoes of those to whom they reach out to bring healing.

We have already shared the definitions of love at the beginning of the book; along with the definitions of both agape and *Unlossable Love*. Not many people who try to understand the definitions of love can view them as only fairy tales that have no basis in reality. If these individuals grow up in dysfunctional homes and environments, the basic drive for love and acceptance that God embeds into all of mankind, that drive will cause them to search for any form of acceptance.

Once this acceptance is obtained, even if this acceptance itself is dysfunctional, people will enslave themselves to those individuals because they are fulfilling (even at the most limited basic level) that need.

A good example of this is the individual who is engaged in a relationship with someone who causes domestic violence and mental anguish in their lives. These individuals know when understanding that the relationship is far from what they ever wanted, yet feel it is the type of relationship that they either deserve because of their low self-esteem or it's the type of relationship that they feel their love can transform that individual into a better person. Often, these types of relationships only create traumas and deeper dysfunctions. The individuals become more broken than ever, and their loss of hope destroys all their dreams of having a happy-ever-after life for themselves.

Look at your own life for a moment: Are you willing to take an honest look at where do you draw your love from and whom you give it to? Is the love that you're looking for and desire the one that you currently have? How did you obtain that love and what did you have to sacrifice for it? Is it/was it worth it for the price that you paid for that love? Who taught you what love is and is not? What misconceptions do you have about love? I understand some of these questions may be tough because it forces us to see what we have and don't have in the means of love in our lives. This is a very scary thing for us to engage in because the findings that we discover may be the exact opposite of the findings we desire.

If we look into the mirror of our soul and see a chasm, do we often try to fill that void with the love that we desire? Again, this is all based upon one's interpretation of what love is and is not, what one's self-value is and is not, and our desire and understanding that we deserve to be loved in the way that we were created to be loved.

I have seen individuals engage in shallow relationships, thinking that the offering of sexual favors and relationships will produce the love that they have always dreamt about. I have seen individuals compromise their belief system totally to the will of those whom they seem to have as their happily ever after and how that individual used and abused this priceless gift. I have seen people who have strong Christian faith compromise that faith to feel desired and loved by someone who can at least fulfill the most limited basic need of love.

As seen, individuals become swindled to believe that the ones who claim that they love have their best intentions and needs—only to find out that this was a manipulation and that the same individuals were doing this to other people in the midst of their intimacy. The betrayal of trust, once exposed, devastates the individual to the point of giving up on not only love but life itself. Some only contemplate suicide while others complete suicide.

These are not exaggerations, and we see examples of this on a regular basis. We hear stories like these from friends and family members. The lack of love and self-worth are the primary contributors to depression, low self-esteem, anxiety, worries, and even suicide. And when you add in other forms of mental illness (sometimes this can be caused by generational traditions and experiences, traumas, and various forms of addictions), people will look in various directions for ways to not feel this emptiness that some have lived in for numerous years.

Speaking from personal experience, when I was a child into my early adulthood, I experienced the journey that I just explained: coming from a dysfunctional family where I was taught that a person is weak to have emotions and that real men don't cry, and that they suck it up when things get tough.

This type of mindset doesn't help an individual to develop healthy relationship-building skills. Obviously, my ability to develop healthy relationships with others was stunted, even though I compromised so much to be loved and accepted by anyone. Each time that I felt that I found that person who would love me for who I am, they would be frightened way by the demands that I never realized that I had in developing strong relationships.

Every time that I would invest myself into a relationship wholeheartedly, we would physically move from that particular city to another (my father was in the military, and we traveled and moved to various places), and the "girlfriend" would dump me for somebody else, or people manipulated me to their desires. It got to the point where all of this caused me to literally reject love: I would refuse to love anyone, to express any form of love, and to accept love from anybody.

After doing this for some time, I became physically ill in a variety of ways (developing ulcers, feeling chest pains even in my teenage years, anger outbursts that would cause me to physically punch inanimate objects—thus hurting myself with bone bruises and sprains, just to name a few). I was depressed, developed the extremely low self-esteem which I still struggle with from time to time today decades later, and I am hyper vigilant on waiting for the next shoe to drop in various relationships.

Once these things began to happen to me, I traced all these incidents back to their origins, which was when I decided to never love again. I was surprised that the lack of love would have such devastation over every aspect of my life, as it did as I went through this time in my life. It was only because of my faith in God, the way that He brought others into my life to restore my hope in love, the way that God directed others to educate me about what love truly is and is not, to open myself to be vulnerable enough to attempt to love once again, that I was able to overcome most of the trauma that I experienced during that time.

I consider myself one of the blessed ones because I didn't do what others have done to cope with their low self-esteem and lack of love. I never turned to drugs or alcohol to give me a false sense of love and acceptance. I never went into shallow relationships to try to trick myself into feeling more popular and accepted than I really was.

I was very fortunate and blessed to begin my faith walk as I began my teenage years. God had strategically placed various individuals of various ages into my life to mentor me and guide me into the love of God, the Father, and to show me how to appropriately love others. I had learned how to not compromise my integrity, my faith, or my quest to find true love.

I can safely say beyond a shadow of a doubt that besides my love for God/Christ/Holy Spirit, the greatest love I have is in my wife, Marsha, to whom, at the time of this writing, I have been married for 38 years joyfully. I have very deep, strong relationships with my best friends, Benny Powell and Bob Ayers, who know me intimately and know every aspect of my life to the present day.

It is said that a man is blessed to have a friend—that is true. I've been blessed with three, as you include Marsha, Benny, and Bob. I have many close loved ones (including the Fosters) that I considered to be precious to me. All of these are a gift from God, and I cherish them with all that I am.

If I would've chased after other avenues of dealing with what I did, I can assure you that I would not be close to the man that I am today. If I would've gone down the same path as those that I've worked with in the mental health field and my pastoral ministry throughout the last 22 years, I believe it would be safe to say that I never would've entered either one of those fields because I would not have listened to God's call on my life.

And I know that I went through what I did in life to prepare me for my callings of being both a pastor and a mental health worker. The experiences that I have had helped me to identify and connect with those whom I would serve and continue to serve. If I would've gone by any other way, it is safe for me to say that I probably would've died years ago at my own hands, if not at the hands of others. It is not a pleasant thing to think about, however, it is the reality of it all. And I've seen this reality in the lives of others: Some of the youth that I've worked with I had buried literally because they involve themselves in activities that they compromised, too, they continued in their waywardness and took their own lives because of the emptiness they felt. I have seen individuals who have taken the lives of others because nobody invested in the love that that individual needed, and they lashed out at the world around them.

For the sake of conversations, let us revisit the 1 Corinthians 13 passage again and lay this as our foundation of what we define love as. Should people use this definition for love, their needs might be fulfilled easier and be longer lasting compared to what the things of this world offer. Love, if it's true, never attempts to be self-seeking and self-fulfilling. We are fulfilled as we pour out the love we seek. It sounds strange, but it is true. Jesus modeled this love to others and in return, they learned and then poured out this deeper and more fulfilling love toward their loved ones. In return, they themselves discovered that the peace and value of this love overpowered the lawlessness of worldly loves. People discovered that this love showed respect, humility, and servanthood, and actually mirrored what Jesus discipling others to share.

In my pastoral counseling, I have done my share of marriage and pre-marriage counseling. I am known to ask these two questions:
- How do you *want* to be loved?
- Are you willing to *teach* one another how you want to be loved?

Many times, these questions throw off the couple because they never had it put to them in this manner. After some thought processing time and conversations, I would then ask the couples these questions:

- How do you want *to love one another*?
- *What is stopping you from loving each other those ways?*

Again, discernment and discussions would follow. This is where the definitions of what they perceived love to be, would be exposed and where honest communication would hopefully be shared. Depending upon responses from one another, the couple would be invited to revisit what began their love for one another and how it has developed over time. If it hadn't developed, we would investigate the reasons why the love relationship has stagnated. Love, if it's true, will take root in our lives and only grow stronger and deeper with one another. And, once real love is established, it never dies. This is evidenced in people who have lost loved ones to death and never stop loving their departed loved ones because of death; that love continues. Should it die, one must ask if this love was based on something different than the definition other than the one shared in this conversation.

When you combine God's agape love, *Unlossable Love,* and the 1 Corinthians 13 passage together, we develop a blueprint in which all other forms of love can begin to establish a foothold on a foundation in which we can customize the loves which we personally desire. It is here where one can say their search for love has been discovered.

WHAT GOD'S UNLOSSABLE LOVE MEANS TO US

Have you ever wondered why love is so important to our existence? The answer was shared in prior chapters: We are created to love and to be loved. Psychologists can testify that the importance of love and value in a human's life is the most important ingredient, which develops stable mental health and relational format. This meets the very basic needs of acceptance.

Without love, the development of social skills and relational skills becomes impaired. Melisa Pita, who writes for CDAclass.org, shares that the loved child has a better chance to become more confident, have better relationships, develop a greater sense of confidence, and are less anxious. Melisa also writes how those children who experience less sense of love are more likely to experience lower self-esteem, have more aggression, and have more behavior problems.

Being created to love and to be loved, we tend to lose focus of this need because we are distracted by the things of this world. As Beatrice and Kenneth have experienced in their fostering, the children whom they receive have had to some degree a lack of positive love and affection; some are severely deprived of love. Both can testify that they have experienced children with multiple behavior problems and extremely low self-esteem.

At the same time, through Beatrice's and Kenneth's stick-to-itiveness, many of these children since have experienced positive love and affection and have seen a notable difference in these children's lives for the better. True, not all have accepted their *Unlossable Love* or any love because they have been so hurt by others rejecting and failing these poor individuals and they use antilove to avoid feeling the devastation of such rejection/loss of love.

The question remains: *What does God's Unlossable Love mean to us?* I could speak in a broad sense or I can speak from personal experiences. I choose the latter as a testimony of God's *Unlossable Love* towards us, and its impact on life—especially when the person chooses to receive this love. It must be noted that even if an individual rejects God's *Unlossable Love,* that doesn't mean God takes it back and withholds it from us; it simply means *we* reject the healing properties that such a love delivers.

As shared in prior chapters, my life had its share of dysfunctions. I became a believer in Christ back in 1977 at a Church of the Nazarene in Confluence, Penn. For the next several years, I was doing a dance between both this world and the spiritual realms (trying to get the best of both worlds, literally). Because of the newly found relationship with God, I began to experience a sense of value, one that I attempted to have filled from my biological father.

My dad was a good man; however, because of his upbringing and a generational curse that transcended from his father's generation, along with other influences, I had not received that value *in the manner I had expected to receive it* (later in life I would discover that it was always there in a sense, but not understood in his manner of showing value towards me). The church and its congregation, by the leading of God's Holy Spirit, began to cultivate in me God's sense of value as not only His servant but as His child. God began to piece together the brokenness which I had experienced. God used my brother David Boyanowski to mentor me in biblical truths and disciplines. I felt like I had some sort of value. Then it happened: David went off to college and moved away and I was left to deal with the family dysfunction all by myself.

My parents and I would eventually move back to Rhode Island (where I was born and raised for most of my early childhood), and I began to attend a Nazarene church in my hometown of Pawtucket. During this time, the dysfunction would yield its ugly head in both my family life and the life of the church. My dad's alcoholism increased because of the pressures in his life and my place in the family was to be the "clean-up crew" after his drunken fits, I would make sure peace was restored to the home and clean up any messes created.

As far as the church, I was able to find great people to assist in mentoring me, and I became a leader within the church. I became the youth group leader and was beginning my studies in the ministry. However, church politics began to be exposed to me, and this began to enrage me!

Because of my past, my experiences have caused me to have (and I continue to have to this day) a passion for the brokenhearted, the neglected, the lost, and rejected. The church went from, in my perception, the Proper Church (one which reflects Jesus' teachings and offers mercy and grace to ALL people) to becoming the Church Proper (a church that is legalistic, self-serving, and exclusive to various individuals because "We don't want such likes . . . "). I had attempted to help change the heart of the congregation by the way I believed God was directing me; however, I found out that I had allowed the Proper Church to change my heart.

As I worked with the youth of the church (mind you, now, I was asked to bring in more youth. Living just outside of Providence, Rhode Island's capital, there is a great amount of inner-city youth that have never been to church, let alone know about the "proper" way to conduct themselves in a church setting), I was informed by the church elders, "You need to get control over these kids, or they are not welcomed here!"

WHAT? This enraged me and I left the church and took a 10-year walk away from the church, religion, and even God Himself. I was rip snorting ticked at God! How could He allow me to have to inflict the pain of rejection on those I was trying to restore? Why would He want me to victimize others the same way those youth and I had experienced rejection?

I must confess; I never gave up on believing in God or gave up on my relationship with Him. I did hold a huge grudge against Him and the Proper Church for those 10 years. My prayer life, studying the Scriptures, and going to church had all passed away. Sure, occasionally I might say a generic prayer, but nothing meaningful. I continued in my waywardness apart from God.

At the same time, God continued with His *Unlossable Love* toward me. Unknown to me, God would utilize this time to mentor me and shape my faith and service to Him. This time "away" from God would show me the true condition of the world: the lack of real love and compassion, the selfishness, and the ways Satan would attack the Church Proper and try to defeat it to get back at God. God would then use the likes of an "outside-the-box" pastor from a United Methodist Church to bring my calling to fruition. His name was Rev. Jack Scott.

In 1990, my mother-in-law was getting remarried to a wonderful man. My wife, Marsha, and our children traveled from Rhode Island to Indiana for the wedding. In a church in Huntertown, Ind., God used Jack Scott to capture my attention. During the rehearsal for the wedding, Jack cracked jokes at the same time he was doing God's work in preparing for the marriage. At first, I thought Jack might have been off his rocker. God also allowed me to see His Spirit working in and through Jack.

After the wedding, the next day, my family attended Jack's church for the first time. Mind you, this was the first church service I had attended in years. I expected to experience the same Church Proper mentality as my former church. What my family and I found was quite the opposite. People greeted us and welcomed us genuinely. One could feel the warmth of God's embrace on our hearts to say, "Welcome home, My child." I didn't know how to respond.

Then came the time for Pastor Jack to enter the service. I didn't know what he was up to, but I do know God had this, especially for my heart. Jack came out wearing an angel costume—not just any angel costume, but a *very* different kind of angel costume . . . Jack's outfit was very dirty and wrinkled, his halo was bent out of shape and crooked. His wings were tattered and ruffled, with some feathers missing. This angel looked like it was run over by a Mack truck and then drugged through the swamps or something like that. I thought for sure, "This guy is a nut job!"

God knew what He was doing because this captivated my attention. This wasn't like any other service I had attended. Then Jack began to share his story. Jack pointed out that in ministry, we all go through battles and struggles. He shared that we often believe that ministries are all organized and clean. Jack continued to share that real ministries call us to battle, that we might get "our feathers ruffled." Life gets dirty, and we will as we assist others to come unto God, and he said that if we truly love others and God, we will gladly engage with the way things of this world tries to hinder the restoration of one's soul and spirit.

Talk about a sledgehammer to the head, *wow!* God opened my eyes to my waywardness, and I recommitted my life to God that day. Within a year's time, my family and I moved to Indiana and began to attend Jack's church.

For the next few years, I would begin to engage in the various ministries of the church. God would restore my brokenness, would call me to use my past experiences to educate evidenced-based practices for connecting with those who are broken, and would call me back into ministry. I *never* thought that God would ever accept me back into His family, let alone to call me to service for Him. God's *Unlossable Love* transformed me and restored me to a deeper and greater love than I had ever known!

I now use this and more as I reach out to the brokenness of the world around us. This is the effect of God's *Unlossable Love* on this writer's soul.

With God, time matters not, and He isn't on anyone's timeframe. What seemed to be a thousand years apart from Him on my behalf, was only a moment for Him. Because of God's *Unlossable Love*, He knows each of us intimately and completely. While I was apart from God, God made a way for me to return to Him. God knows that I am a person of peculiar interests, so God used a peculiar pastor to reach me and led me back to Christ and my calling. God is now using me to do the same for others.

Because of God's intimacy with each of us, He knows the perfect place, timing, circumstances, and even storms in our lives to capture our attention. He never forces Himself on us but allows us the choice to be found. In this, God shows value and dignity towards us. He models for us the approach which not only works the best but also is less intrusive. Love is supportive, compassionate, and enduring. It grants the one in need of it whatever time is needed to complete its task of restoration and healing. A single act of love can harvest a hundredfold when allowed to take root in our souls.

What does God's *Unlossable Love* mean to us? I know what it means to me. You might differ from my response. Your experiences and beliefs are not the same as mine because we each are uniquely made. God's love towards us remains the same: in vastness, in expression, in grace and in mercy. It endures forever and even Hell has no power over it. I know the potential that it has to impact life, especially a life that has been broken and is in need of healing.

God's *Unlossable Love* means that there is a love for everyone that will never give up on you and will always seek to make you the very best version of who you are. This love is the ultimate love because it is God directly. When a person accepts God's love in any form, they are transformed and are no longer what they once were. When an individual is touched by true love, they are no longer the same forever. That love empowers them and motivates them to become the very best that they can possibly strive for; not to earn the ability to keep that love but because of that love they are motivated and can see their potential.

Speaking for myself (although I know many will agree with me), I know intimately all my mistakes, sins, and poor choices. I know the depths of the darkness that I can possess from time to time, and I know how depraved my mind can be.

God knows all of this and at the same time, He sees my potential, my true heart's desire, and how much suffering I have when I trick myself into those dark places and He loves me anyway. He knows that the darkness is not the true reflection of my heart or of my desires. Because God created me and knows me intimately, He continues to mentor me and love me and seeks to have intimacy with me. When anybody, especially God, loves me like that, I cherish that relationship because they also chose to cherish me. That is life-changing and that is what God's agape/*Unlossable Love* does for us. I know the impact that this is had on my life and how it is continually transforming me to become a person after God's own heart.

If you would like to experience this for yourself, God is eagerly awaiting to fulfill your needs and to love you unconditionally and wholeheartedly. He is that missing piece that drives each of us most of our lives to try to find and fulfill. It is our relationship with the Holy God that brings us the ultimate *Unlossable Love* that we strive for and need. Yes, we may find *Unlossable Love* in others and we ourselves may become agents for this love; however, to share it we must first experience it. Regardless of what your choice may be, remember that we already have this love from God. All we must do is accept.

IS MANKIND CAPABLE OF UNLOSSABLE LOVE?

We have just shared that man can experience God's *Unlossable Love* because He is that love and He desires to have all mankind receive and embrace this love. The title of this chapter asks a very good question: *Is Mankind Capable of Unlossable Love?*

We hinted at the answer in previous chapters that man can be capable of *Unlossable Love*; however, to develop this love will feel like an uphill battle in which you are pushing the massive stone to the mountaintop. *Unlossable Love* is something that would take total commitment, and ongoing perseverance during times when you feel weak or completely drained of love, involves an ongoing connection with the individual(s) that you are modeling this for, and the most important aspect of it is that you receive this love and understand it fully before trying to live this out.

If you have not experienced *Unlossable Love* and understand the importance of how this love can revitalize a person's spirit and soul, how can you teach this properly? This is where we have to rely on God being able to teach us about this love, to accept and own this love, as God desires us to, and then to model it to the world that needs it most.

We know and understand that this is a huge undertaking and that this is asking a lot of us who engage in *Unlossable Love*; that is because the stakes are high: It is not only the spiritual life of the individual(s), but it is also the mental and emotional health, and possibly even the physical health (for those who are suffering emotionally and mentally, suicidal ideation could become a very real sought after outcome when a person doesn't feel valued/love/accepted). And if you are one of the individuals who may feel this way, you know exactly what I am referring to. You understand the vast void that lies within your soul, and you yearn for acceptance and love. You know the deep darkness that can overtake you with that flicker of light absent within your soul.

This is why it is vitally important for each of us to know and understand that our commitment to this love and sharing it with others should be the same type of commitment that God has given us through both His agape/*Unlossable Love*. For those of us who have received this love and understand it, we not only know how valuable it is but also understand the healing power that it has for everyone who desires it.

In speaking with Beatrice, I asked her to share with me how she was able to personally develop *Unlossable Love* in her life. I had also inquired what made her desire to adapt this into her life and what steps, if any, did she take to infuse into her personal life. This is her response:

I believe that God developed this over time in my life. I have a performance personality; I thrive at doing things exceedingly well and I hate failure. As a child, I was very well behaved, I thought that the better behaved I was the more I would be liked/loved by my parents and others. I carried that same mentality into work and marriage. The positive about this personality is that I am exceptional at what I do and all I seek is praise. The negative about it is that I only feel loved when I feel that I have deserved it, I do not allow myself to make mistakes and when I do I am very hard on myself. When I became a Christian, I carried this same mentality into my walk with Christ. In 2018, I "failed" God, or so I thought. I spent days wondering if my decision just cost me the love of my Savior. When I finally approached Him in prayer, I realized that He was still there waiting with open arms, waiting for me, ready to love me. My performance driven personality was shattered at the moment because in my mind, I didn't deserve love. At that moment, I experienced what God was already shaping and forming into my life through my dear friend Meredith.

A couple of years earlier God brought me my dear friend, Meredith, who did not share my personality, but she was similar because she was taught that her worth/acceptance/love was directly related to her performance as a child, Christian, and person. As she and I began our relationship, she shared with me the baggage she carried of not being loved or accepted because of her life choices; she carried deep scars. I felt like God wanted me to do the opposite of what she expected and make a commitment to her as a person that I would always be there for her, no matter her decisions or actions. This is a commitment that is easy to say but harder to live. I knew that I would be involved in her life for years; however long it took to help repair those scars. Over time and through many hard moments, Meredith realized that my love for her was not wavering or leaving and that I was someone that she could call on in a moment's notice for help. My love for her is not perfect; I have made my share of mistakes but it's still there. God's perfect love for Meredith was being shown to her through me; as a result, Meredith saw Jesus and decided to follow Him.

After I experienced my "failure" and God's love through that time, I realized that God was showing me a first-hand experience of what He was already calling me to do with Meredith. I was able to understand better and see the magnitude of receiving this love and how it can change a person. I already had a God-given drive to love Meredith like this but now I felt like this was more than Meredith, it needed to be shared with everyone.—Beatrice

I would like to share some insights into Beatrice's responses. As you begin to read the first paragraph of her response, Beatrice shares this isn't a quick fix, and one cannot instantly develop it in a short period of time. As you read her response, Beatrice shares, in her vulnerability, some very personal details and struggles that she faced. It is clear that Beatrice didn't have any foreknowledge or understanding of what *Unlossable Love* was or that such a thing ever existed. She shared how thought processes can be insecure and sometimes even irrational to make one believe things that are not true or that things can't be changed.

How many of us can identify with this? (How many of us are willing to admit such a thing?) It is very common for people to feel that their identity is based upon their performance and that acceptance only comes with positive performance. The problem with this mindset, as indicated by Beatrice, is that our self-worth is all based upon what others think or feel and not based on our own understanding of ourselves and our understanding of our true value to God and others.

Looking at this through God's eyes, His agape/*Unlossable Love* isn't based upon performance; it simply exists because God created it and freely gives it to us. As a person begins to be introduced to *Unlossable Love*, we understand that this love is the divine answer to God's agape love, which has nothing to do with any sort of performance that we have committed ourselves to, it simply exists because of God's good pleasure towards us. When both of these loves are combined together and intertwined to where one cannot be separated from the other, we as humans can hopefully begin to stop using our performances as qualifiers to love of any sort.

Another insight I would like to draw your attention to is what Beatrice has shared about the commitment that one needs to make towards the individuals they are trying to introduce this *Unlossable Love* to. In Beatrice's statement, she shares, "This is a commitment that is easy to say but harder to live. I knew that I would be involved in her life for years; however long it took to help repair those scars."

I do fully agree with Beatrice that is one pledge to be there for somebody, we should do it with all of our beings and do our very best to live up to that which we have committed to. At the same time, in the last part of Beatrice's statement, she commented " . . . to help repair those scars." Try as we may, we are not qualified enough to have the ability to repair scars, whether they be emotional, mental, or spiritual scars.

Psychologists and therapists cannot erase the scars; they can only assist in reducing the pain's effectiveness to immobilize us from progressing on with our lives. They can help us to understand what has caused the pain and to be able to equip us on how to deal with the pain. The scars will forever be part of our lives, no matter how far we tried to bury them or ignore them. This isn't to discount Beatrice's desire to bring healing and restoration; this is what we're trying to do with everybody that we love and care for. This is about how God's agape/*Unlossable Love* equips us to be used by Him to bring healing and restoration to the individuals we reach out to.

In 2008, I was involved in an auto accident *that should have* taken my life: I struck a tree going 55 mph, which broke every rib in my body with the exception of one, broke my neck, broke my leg, my hand went through the windshield, and I had a broken nose and several lacerations on my body. It goes without saying, I received several gnarly scars from this accident. Yes, I could have several more procedures that would remove the physical scars on my body, but this would not change the emotional and mental scars that I have from the accident. These will be and are forever part of me. I may be able to reduce some of the trauma effects, but I will always have an impact from the trauma. No amount of therapy will be able to remove this from who I am today. This is where God was able to transform my focus from being a victim to becoming victorious over my circumstances.

God showed me through His love how to embrace my scars and to use them as a positive reminder versus the negative reminders that most people believe that to be. As people look at my physical scars, they make comments like, "That must've been a very painful event for you!" "Boy, you're lucky! You could have been killed in that wreck!" And my personal favorite, "How did you ever survive the accident?"

In my responses to the statements, especially about the scars, I was able to share God's insight into my situation: "When you see scars, you see the pain that I must have suffered. You focus on the hurt and what should have happened to me. I look at the same scars and I see the tremendous healing that has taken place because of God's providence in my life and His great love toward me. You look at the scars and can only think of the trauma that occurred. I look at those same scars and see the deliverance of what should have overtaken my life and how God preserved my life in one of the darkest moments of not only my life; but also that of my family's and loved ones' lives."

Once people hear this statement, they begin to think about and ponder how someone like myself is thinking along those lines. Simply put, because of God. I am very much human and there are times when I have flawed thinking and irrational thoughts. Even in the midst of that accident, I did not fear death, becoming an invalid, or any other fears because I knew that my life was in the hands of a loving God who love me unconditionally and I had total faith in His love towards me. This allowed my attitude and focus to not only be a positive one, but God was able to use me in various circumstances and other people's lives as I was healing in every manner of the word.

Just like Beatrice, isn't it just like each of us desire to remove the pain in the scars from those whom we love? And if this is so, why can we not do that for ourselves? In the same way that we look at others and desire this, we must also look within ourselves to desire this for ourselves.

How many of us are carrying around mental, emotional, and spiritual baggage that we would love to let go of, but cannot because we deem ourselves unworthy? As we shared earlier, it is important for us to know when to understand exactly what this *Unlossable Love* is by experiencing it to its fullest potential, accepting it, and then growing from it.

As Beatrice has shared with her friend Meredith, "As she and I began our relationship, she shared with me the baggage she carried of not being loved or excepted because of her life choices; she carried deep scars. I felt like God wanted me to do the opposite of what she expected and make a commitment to her as a person that I would always be there for her, no matter her decisions or actions. This is a commitment that is easy to say but harder to live. I knew that I would be involved in her life for years; however long it took to help repair those scars. Over time and through many hard moments, Meredith realized that my love for her was not wavering or leaving and that I was someone that she could call at a moment's notice for help."

Beatrice knew and understood because of her connectedness with God what God required of her to reach Meredith. Beatrice had to show by example that she was not like the rest of the world, which compounded Meredith's low self-image and acceptance of herself. Beatrice shares this in the last paragraph of her quote.

It should also be noted that before Beatrice attempted to share God's *Unlossable Love* with Meredith, Beatrice and Meredith had a foundation of love established. As Beatrice was able to introduce Meredith to God's love, it became abundantly apparent to Meredith that she finally found somebody to be able to begin to trust enough to follow their lead.

This trust is a key component for man to be able to live out God's *Unlossable Love* in others. If we have an established relationship with an individual and that relationship is a healthy one, this allows God to be able to use us in a more powerful way than if we were first meeting the individual and attempting to educate them in what God's love truly is. If a person does not trust us, they will not listen to us; regardless of how good it sounds or makes them feel.

People are not looking for words; they are looking for actions and results. If our lives do not reflect that which we are teaching, people will see that within a moment's time and ignore us. However, if an individual is able to build up trust between themselves and another person, both are more receptive to learning from one another. This trust enables us to put into action something that is tangible for the other person to receive, understand, and utilize. Allow me to give you a biblical example:

> *On the evening of that day, the first day of the week, the doors being locked where the disciples were for fear of the Jews, Jesus came and stood among them and said to them, "Peace be with you." When he had said this, he showed them his hands and his side. Then the disciples were glad when they saw the Lord. Jesus said to them again, "Peace be with you. As the Father has sent me, even so I am sending you." And when he had said this, he breathed on them and said to them, "Receive the Holy Spirit. If you forgive the sins of any, they are forgiven them; if you withhold forgiveness from any, it is withheld.*
>
> *Now Thomas, one of the twelve, called the Twin, was not with them when Jesus came. So the other disciples told him, "We have seen the Lord." But he said to them, "Unless I see in his hands the mark of the nails, and place my finger into the mark of the nails, and place my hand into his side, I will never believe."*
>
> *Eight days later, his disciples were inside again, and Thomas was with them. Although the doors were locked, Jesus came and stood among them and said, "Peace be with you." Then he said to Thomas, "Put your finger here, and see my hands, and put out your hand, and place it in my side. Do not disbelieve but believe." Thomas answered him, "My Lord and my God!" Jesus said to him, "Have you believed because you have seen me? Blessed are those who have not seen and yet have believed." (John 20:19–29)*

Just like Thomas, we want proof of the reality that we profess. If we cannot prove to others that this is real, they will not believe us. (Even if we have this evidence, there are still those who will deny it because they may feel that it's not for them for whatever reason.) The women and the disciples all testified to Thomas about seeing the risen Christ. Thomas refused to believe such an impossible event could have taken place.

How much are we like Thomas and cannot conceive the possibility of what God can do? In looking at our own lives, we consider ourselves broken beyond repair, unlovable because of the numerous sins and wrongs that we have done and we cannot forgive ourselves for (please note that I shared that *we ourselves* believe and not what God believes). And take note in this particular passage that before Thomas could even say a single word that Christ was able to answer his statement that Thomas had made out of earshot of Jesus one week earlier. At that very moment, when Thomas received clarity, Thomas was able to conceive and believe everything that the Disciples and the women were able to share.

Again, review the words that Beatrice was able to share with Meredith: " . . . I realize that God was showing me a firsthand experience of what he was really calling me to do with Meredith. I was able to understand better and see the magnitude of receiving this love and how it can change a person. I already had a God-given drive to love Meredith like this, but now I felt like this was more than Meredith, it needed to be shared with everyone."

I agree wholeheartedly with Beatrice in this statement.

In my continued investigation with Beatrice on the various questions I had asked of her, she shares a beautiful example of how *Unlossable Love* needs to be administered to the people who need it most to assist them to overcome the various traumas and obstacles that prevent them from experiencing God's love and the love of others in their lives:

Is Mankind Capable of Unlossable Love?

I recently sat and talked with my daughter's boyfriend, Steve. He was struggling in their relationship because of the effects of her trauma-filled life. My daughter has trust issues with men, stemming from her childhood trauma. As a result, she struggles to trust Steve despite his actions and words. As we talked, I explained to him her trauma and how it affects her and her relationship with him. I explained that his words would not be enough to gain her trust, he would have to commit a lifetime to her, of actions. I explained Unlossable Love to him, I encouraged him to look at her as a Mount Everest expedition. One that would take years of planning and attempts before gaining the summit. I told him, "One day she will trust you, it might be in 1 month, 1 year or 15 years or it might not ever happen. You will have little "wins" and hard "losses" along the way. Just keep loving and forgiving her." I hope that he takes that advice and runs with it, I hope that their relationship flourishes, but time will tell.—Beatrice

Once again, being very vulnerable and transparent, Beatrice shares an example of the commitment that a person must have to present this love to others. People will respond to it unquestionably; however, sometimes it may not be in the way that we hope for.

Beatrice shared this with Steve, and she was able to give a history of what happened because of the trauma-filled life in his girlfriend's personal experience. She shared with Steve that if he is able to reach her and prove to her the ability to trust men can be restored, he would have to become the reality for her by just not his words, but his actions as well.

Beatrice shared with Steve that this is a total commitment, an ongoing commitment, a commitment that will have its ups and downs, victories and failures, and even the possibilities that it may not come about the way that he hoped for. I love her statement when she instructs

Unlossable Love

Steve, too, "Just keep loving and forgiving her." This is the perfect example of God's agape/*Unlossable Love* which he imparts to every one of us all the time and every time we need it.

To piggyback off what Beatrice has shared, this is the way that I tried to live now that I know that what I've been trying to share all my life is actually the *Unlossable Love* that I have longed for and searched for all of my life. I have tried to become everything that I look for in the realm of love and relationship with both God and man. Because of being introduced to the phrase by Beatrice, I now have a name for that which I searched for. I also now can express it because I've experienced it not only from God, but also from my wife, Marsha, and the rest of my family, extremely close friends whom God has brought into my life, and I am able to begin to love myself in the same fashion because of God. I am also able to live this out in the lives of everybody that I know and to assist them to turn from their "Thomas stance" (only believe in after seeing) and to bring God's love to everyone who allows me to humble privilege and honor of living this out through God and because of God. I am witness to how God uses His love to transform lives; one of which is my own life.

Is man capable of *Unlossable Love*? Absolutely! If one is willing to put in the time and effort into their own life and the lives of others, trust in and rely on God in following His lead through the Holy Spirit, nothing is impossible! Speaking from experience, it is absolutely worth every ounce of my being that is put into this to be able to see the results of what God has done in my own life and what God has done through His love. I am positive you will feel the same way once you experience it for yourself.

> *My hope and goal is that God uses my family and our love as an encouragement to others, not with our words, but with our actions. Our mentorship is through example; people watching us*

live our lives as we feel God is calling us to. My only struggle has been myself. I get in my own way. I am selfish and I want to do what I want to do. I don't want to get hurt again. I do not want to watch someone make bad choices. I do not want to love this person who has hurt me. Unlossable Love is not about me. Unlossable love is about God's love for us. Unlossable love is about others.—Beatrice

UNLOSSABLE LOVE AND TAINTED PASTS

Unlossable Love sounds good; at least for those whom we believe *deserve* such love. What about those who have hurt us, abused us, and left us for dead (emotionally and mentally; and sadly, sometimes physically)? Looking inwardly, as we look at our faults and failures, are poor choices and decisions, can we move past our tainted pasts to obtain a clear and beautiful future? That is the trillion-dollar question asked by many.

Being a pastor for the last 22 years, one of the questions that I hear repeatedly is this: "Pastor John, I know God is all about forgiveness, turning the other cheek and all that; however, how do you forgive someone who has done some very bad things to you?"

I will not bore you with spiritual clichés the Church Proper might spew out. I also will not share psychological babble that a therapist may share. To do so would only insult your intelligence and your capability for trust. To be transparent with you, I sometimes wonder the same thing, and I'm supposed to be a pastor who lives out forgiveness. Because I'm very much human and how my past is tainted, I would have to admit that I sometimes struggle with this very question and living out what I'm about to teach.

To be able to teach this, we must first have an understanding of what is right and what is wrong. It is easy to say that you have a clear understanding of the two and you may have some concept of this. The real question is: *By whose standard* are you using it? This is where it gets tricky. The reason for this statement is that we go by our spiritual standards found within God's Holy Word (the Bible) and the leading of the Holy Spirit, we have one standard. (This is based upon the Christian faith for the purpose of this book.) If we go by another religion's standards, this will differ. If we go by the standard that there is no belief in God/deity, there is yet another standard. And if we go based upon the worldview standard that sin does not exist, there is yet that other standard. As stated earlier, I'm approaching this through the Christian point of view.

The concept between what is right and what is wrong varies from one belief system to the other. In the Christian faith, what is right and what is wrong is established in the book of Genesis when we look at the story of Adam and Eve in the Garden. God gave man one simple rule to follow:

> *When no bush of the field was yet in the land and no small plant of the field had yet sprung up—for the L*ORD *God had not caused it to rain on the land, and there was no man to work the ground, and a mist was going up from the land and was watering the whole face of the ground— then the L*ORD *God formed the man of dust from the ground and breathed into his nostrils the breath of life, and the man became a living creature. And the L*ORD *God planted a garden in Eden, in the east, and there he put the man whom he had formed. And out of the ground the L*ORD *God made to spring up every tree that is pleasant to the sight and good for food. The tree of life was in the midst of the garden, and the tree of the knowledge of good and evil.*
>
> *A river flowed out of Eden to water the garden, and there it divided and became four rivers. The name of the first is the Pishon. It is the one that flowed around the whole land of Havilah, where there is gold. And the gold of that land is good; bdellium and onyx stone are there. The name of the second river is the Gihon. It is the*

> one that flowed around the whole land of Cush. And the name of the third river is the Tigris, which flows east of Assyria. And the fourth river is the Euphrates.
>
> The LORD God took the man and put him in the garden of Eden to work it and keep it. And the LORD God commanded the man, saying, "You may surely eat of every tree of the garden, but of the tree of the knowledge of good and evil you shall not eat, for in the day that you eat of it you shall surely die." (Genesis 2:5–17)

God gave Adam free rein over all of creation on the earth apart from one: to not eat of the tree of knowledge of good and evil. One simple rule to follow. If God did not want Adam to eat the tree, why would he place it in the Garden of Eden? Because for man to have free will, the man had to have a choice. If there is no choice, there is no ability to have free will.

God has given all of mankind the ability to have free will and to be able to make choices for themselves. Along with the ability to have free choice comes the responsibility for that choice. God clearly shared with Adam what the consequence would be for disobeying His one directive. As you read beyond this Scripture passage for several more verses, we see Adam and Eve using their ability to have free will to make a choice that would affect all of mankind forever more. Their choice to eat from the tree of knowledge of good and evil caused the division between God and man. The serpent (Satan disguised as the serpent) was able to convince Eve to partake of the fruit and Eve shared it with Adam. Thus, this became a sin to man. All of mankind has struggled with sin from that point on throughout all of the ages and will continue to struggle with it until Christ returns.

There are those who believe that if they do not believe in God, there is no sin. If there is no sin, there is no responsibility for their actions. They are able to do whatever they want to whomever they want whenever they want. They take advantage of not knowing the true difference between right and wrong in the eyes of God to do whatever they want in their own eyes. The last sentence in the book of Judges in the Bible shares this haunting reality when there is no accountability for someone's actions: *"In those days there was no king in Israel. Everyone did what was right in his own eyes." (Judges 21:25)*

In this example, the people did whatever was right in their own eyes because there were no boundaries that could be enforced and upheld. In today's world, we see the effects of such a mindset. For many, if you are brought up with this understanding from the time you were born until the present, it is understandable how the past is tainted by their present and possible future.

I believe there are those who truly don't know the difference between right and wrong in the biblical sense/faith-based sense because religion isn't an important part of their lives. Equally noted, the same can be said of the moral decline in society follows the Judges passage because the family unit is dissolving; marriages are on the decline, single parents are on the rise, the absenteeism of fathers in the home is also increasing, people are living together and are not committing to family structures; thus, avoiding accountability. These and more contribute to the mindset of Judges: no accountability, no boundaries, and structures which lead to no limits as to what man will do to get what he wants. It matters not as to what effect this has on others; so long as their desires are met to their satisfaction.

Apart from these, we ourselves also wrestle with tainted pasts. If we confess to being believers in God/Jesus Christ/Holy Spirit; we can't avoid this knowledge. The Holy Spirit reveals to the believers that sin is real and our need for a Savior. As this revelation comes, guilt accompanies this because we now know that we have created sin in our lives, and we begin to assess how this has affected others. When we see the effects and understand how *we have created these impacts*, we become our own judge, prosecutor, and executioner. We find ourselves guilty, sentence ourselves to the "fullest extent" of the law, and our "execution" is a lifetime of guilt and shame without a chance of forgiveness from ourselves. Yes, we might receive grace and mercy from God and others, but we refuse to forgive our tainted past. We convince ourselves that there's nothing we can do to "make up" for what we did. Especially when we have wronged someone we love, the solitary confinement of guilt and shame becomes every time we take another breath. We try to get past this by changing our actions, trying to base our worth on works more than on who we are in Christ. Yet, the memories continue to convict us repeatedly. This causes us to lose more self-love and value for ourselves, so we try harder to rise above these and work even more for our redemption.

Unlossable Love now becomes even more important here! This is where this love can become the freedom fighter we need to remind us that God allows us to forgive ourselves if we truly desire to. Our past doesn't have to define us. God reminds us that His agape/*Unlossable Love* refines us to remove the impurities. The memories remain to remind us how our wrongdoings have wounded and destroyed that which we love so now we can choose to avoid repeating the same behaviors, actions, and attitudes that had led us to the isolation we condemned ourselves to.

God's love has pardoned us and frees us to move on from it. To accomplish this within ourselves, we *must* model God's agape/*Unlossable Love* inwardly. As stated in earlier chapters, for us to effectively execute God's love towards others, we must experience and adopt this love in and for ourselves. This becomes a living testimony to how His love can and does transform a tainted past into a beautiful work of grace for all to witness for themselves. This is what draws others to the presence of God Almighty and allows restoration of fellowship with the Creator.

Unlossable Love and Tainted Pasts

You might be saying, "You *truly* don't understand my situation! If you only knew the past, I have. . . . " True. I might not know your situation and past; however, I know our God and Who He is . . . I know the Creator of all has the capability and freely gives this to each of us to release our sinful and flawed thoughts and actions and to transform us into new creations:

Therefore, knowing the fear of the Lord, we persuade others. But what we are is known to God, and I hope it is known also to your conscience. We are not commending ourselves to you again but giving you cause to boast about us, so that you may be able to answer those who boast about outward appearance and not about what is in the heart. For if we are beside ourselves, it is for God; if we are in our right mind, it is for you. For the love of Christ controls us because we have concluded this: that one has died for all, therefore all have died; and he died for all, that those who live might no longer live for themselves but for him who for their sake died and was raised.

*From now on, therefore, we regard no one according to the flesh. Even though we once regarded Christ according to the flesh, we regard him thus no longer. Therefore, if anyone is in Christ, he is a **new creation**. The old has passed away; behold, the **new** has come. All this is from God, who through Christ reconciled us to himself and gave us the ministry of reconciliation; that is, in Christ God was reconciling the world to himself, not counting their trespasses against them, and entrusting to us the message of reconciliation. Therefore, we are ambassadors for Christ, God making his appeal through us. We implore you on behalf of Christ, be reconciled to God. For our sake he made him to be sin who knew no sin, so that in him we might become the righteousness of God. (2 Corinthians 5:11–21)*

Please read and reread this passage several times. Allow it to penetrate deep within your soul. Ponder the wonders of grace and restoration this can bring if we accept it for ourselves. I understand that all who are reading this book might not be believers or have a faith system and this might only sound like empty words. Even if I share with you that I am a living testimony to this truth (which I am professing), you might have doubts. Because of tainted pasts, traumas, and loss of trust, I get it. I was once where you are now . . . not knowing what to believe or whom to believe.

I once believed that I didn't deserve forgiveness from anyone because of the pain and hurt I personally caused and created. I have tortured myself time and time again in hopes of some sort of "restitution" of my soul through my works. I tried self-justification, which failed miserably. I ignored my guilt by believing if I just turned things around that my good works would surpass my failures and I would change my image; that only gave me the appearance of better self-esteem all the while I secretly suffered my self-execution emotionally. Does it sound familiar?

Tainted pasts only have as much control over our lives as we give them permission to have. We have complete control over how we respond to not only our circumstances but also to the ways we respond/react to these. This leads me to this question; one that Jesus would often ask those who sought His healing touch: "Do you want to be healed?" Some people don't know just how much they need healing because they can't feel the state they are in; their tainted past has left them paralyzed and numb. Like cancer, it silently destroys from within and if left unnoticed, death will follow.

Are you feeling numb or paralyzed and long to feel again? Are you allowing your past to taint your present? God's *Unlossable Love* longs to unchain you to be free to release yourself to forgive yourself and finally deal with the tainted past you are held captive by. Satan will try to convince you that you are unforgiveable; however, God knows that's a lie! Come forth and be free once and for all!

UNLOSSABLE LOVE TOWARDS OTHER

Now that we have dealt with *our tainted pasts*, how about others' past histories? Can we overcome what we believe is unforgivable in others? Now, before you answer, think hard and deeply! Allow me to throw a few curveballs at you to get your blood boiling:
- People who have caused us/loved one's great traumas.
- People whose actions had caused the death of someone we love
- People who have caused us great loss and have no remorse or repentance for their action
- Individuals who belittle us/loved ones.
- Individuals/groups that believe differently than we do.
- Individuals who have different belief systems
- Racial differences
- Political differences
- Known biases.
- Economic differences (either higher or lower income than your own)
- Authors of injustices
- Divorces
- Foster Care issues—being removed from the home and placed with foster families (blaming the parents or siblings which might have caused the removal because of behaviors and actions not your own)

I could go on; but you get where I am going. These situations easily cause one to want to cast them into Hell after they suffer ten times as much of the suffering they caused us/others. This is where the rubber meets the road: can we forgive their tainted pasts (or even their present)? Will we allow God's agape/*Unlossable Love* to be extinguished by our biases and prejudices? Are we willing to offer the same grace we desire from others and God?

If we seek relief from our tainted past, it is not only our duty to offer this to others, but it is also our humble honor to assist God in the restoration of others. If we follow the voice of God, we are called to become more like Christ and less like us. Christ gave us examples that are recorded in the Scriptures. His Disciples are perfect examples. Paul the Apostle is another. We must pray for others the same things we seek for ourselves. This is what brings God joy and our examples of His healing touch on our lives.

I had listed the examples I shared because when we are confronted by these and other examples, one or more will cause our blood to boil. We see daily how injustices take place and those perpetrators of such despicable things never get the justice *we think they deserve*. We want them to know *exactly* how they made us feel, the depth of the pain we are suffering, and for it to last at least as long as what we are/will experience. I can remember how it felt and from time to time it revisits me and tries to cause me discomfort and pain.

Even with these extreme examples that have been provided, how many times do we hold people accountable with consequences more than they deserve? I'm sure that you can agree that you have witnessed at some point in your life that someone might have done something wrong and the punishment for that wrong was complete overkill. How often do we provide overkill to those who offend us? Why is it that we demand more retribution than what it is called for? One theory I have is that we want to make sure, beyond a shadow of a doubt, that that person never desires to repeat the offense.

Where does *Unlossable Love* fit in with this mindset? Obviously, it doesn't. Yes, there is a need for natural consequences to take place so that we may learn from our mistakes. It is quite necessary to add God's agape/*Unlossable Love* so that grace may be added for this to become a teachable moment rather than the hardening of the heart. Most of these individuals involved already have a hardened heart and it needs to be softened through the mercy of God and His love. When we add our own human consequences and desires for harsh penalties without mercy, the heart becomes even more densely hardened.

In my work in the mental health field, I have worked with parents, foster parents, foster children, siblings, and more who all have opinions and struggle with those who have caused their issues. For some, there is forgiveness. For most, resentment, anger, rage, abandonment, not being valued, loss of love and respect from those who are "supposed to be there for them," anxieties, rejection, and more fill the hearts like the lead weight of an anchor tossed into a bottomless abyss. Because of the deep traumas that were caused by their parents or siblings and being thrust into the great unknown of the foster care system or having to work with mental health, there is great resentment because they feel that they are being forced into this and that they have no control over their circumstance and situation. Therefore, it is conceivable for individuals in those predicaments to have such feelings toward what they are currently going through. This doesn't make their actions correct, it simply means in their own minds they justify their thoughts and feelings, and responses.

Think about a time when you had caused trauma or a negative impact on somebody's life: how did it make you feel? Hopefully, there was a sense of guilt or remorse that quickly followed the incident. In that circumstance, what was the outcome? Don't answer too quickly; please think deeply about how you frame your answer. Did those individuals forgive you, and if so, how was that forgiveness granted to you? What was it about them and your relationship with that individual that allowed you forgiveness for your actions?

If you did not receive forgiveness from that individual, how did/does this impact you? Why do you think they did not offer you forgiveness? Love. If the individual(s) forgave you, love was the motivator and the bridge to be able to extend forgiveness. Maybe that love was not towards you but may be a direct reflection of God's love towards you, a love for others that you have impacted, and they chose to love them enough to forgive you to end their pain and suffering by bringing peace to the relationship. It may have been even the love towards you that moves them to love. If they chose not to love you, they obviously won't grant you that love *until they are moved by love* to offer and grant you the forgiveness you seek.

Here's why it is so important to extend love and forgiveness toward others: love transforms the person who might have never experienced it to become the greatest advocate for love. Perfect examples from literature are The Grinch and Ebenezer Scrooge. Both individuals had tainted pasts and traumas that contributed to their current bitterness and disconnection from others. Their experiences with rejection led them to become hard-hearted. Most people either hated or feared them. In each of their stories, a small child (Cindy-Lou Who in *How the Grinch Stole Christmas* and Tiny Tim for *A Christmas Carol*) became the changing agent for their hard hearts to melt. The townspeople had already cast them aside socially and deemed them outcasts. But through the eyes of these little ones, both Grinch and Scrooge discovered the errors of their ways, made amends, and became far better restored than they ever imagined! Can you now see how just one person believing in them transformed and restored their broken lives?

Here is where we discuss spirituality. An often-overlooked aspect of brokenness lies beneath the soul which is caused by the lack of spirituality or the neglect of our spiritual selves. People are very aware of the mental and emotional impacts; however, to deny our spirituality is to forfeit a valuable tool in holistic healing and restoration. A doctor wouldn't perform an operation without the use of a scalpel to make the necessary incisions. Healing would never take place. If God's *Unlossable Love* is to bring total healing, it must be applied where it is needed most. Like a doctor, they can treat many of the symptoms, but unless they discover the core problem, the patient could bleed out and die.

Jesus, in His ministry, would meet every aspect of the individual's needs:

- Physically—From feeding the hungry to raising people from the dead, Jesus met the physical needs because He knew people are distracted from everything else when they are concerned about how that need might (if even possible) be met. By meeting the physical needs, Jesus had their undivided attention to address other needs.
- Mentally—Jesus was and remains passionate about our mental needs. Jesus would remind people to "not worry," "cast your cares upon the LORD," "peace, be still," and other ways to prevent or heal mental anguish. Jesus made sure that the people had a clear understanding of what he was trying to teach and make sure that each was mentally capable to retain what he was trying to teach.
- Emotionally—"Fear not . . . ," "Do not be afraid . . . ," "Don't let your anger cause you to sin . . . " are a few ways Jesus addresses emotional distress. Even when Jesus wept, Jesus had the assurance of knowing that emotions are a true normal feeling; however, a person should not live by emotions because emotions sometimes blind us from seeing the possibilities and the realities that lie ahead.
- Spiritually—After dealing with all the prior needs, Jesus *always* addresses the spiritual needs of connecting with God, finding forgiveness, and having trust/faith in God and His capabilities.

I remind you now, Jesus did this for those individuals which abused Him most (the guards who nailed Him to the cross after beating Him), who betrayed Him (Judas), those who abandoned Him (His disciples) and those who worshipped Him one day and later that same week had condemned Him to death. Jesus was still able to impart agape/ *Unlossable Love* to all of creation. Jesus took time to share God's love with all because we all need that love. It is this love that each of us is called to give to everyone we meet, develop a relationship with, even those whom society deems deplorable. His results are countless and are recorded in the Scriptures and in our hearts.

If you are willing to be used by God, He can/will use us to bring His love to others. This will, in turn, bring salvation, restoration, peace, and value to the very least of these:

> *The word reached the king of Nineveh, and he arose from his throne, removed his robe, covered himself with sackcloth, and sat in ashes. And he issued a proclamation and published through Nineveh, "By the decree of the king and his nobles: Let neither man nor beast, herd nor flock, taste anything. Let them not feed or drink water, but let man and beast be covered with sackcloth, and let them call out mightily to God. Let everyone turn from his evil way and from the violence that is in his hands. Who knows? God may turn and relent and turn from his fierce anger, so that we may not perish."*
>
> *When God saw what they did, how they turned from their evil way, God relented of the disaster that he had said he would do to them, and he did not do it.*
>
> *But it displeased Jonah exceedingly, and he was angry. And he prayed to the LORD and said, "O LORD, is not this what I said when I was yet in my country? That is why I made haste to flee to Tarshish; for I knew that you are a gracious God and merciful, slow to anger and abounding in steadfast love, and relenting from disaster. Therefore now, O LORD, please take my life from me, for it is better for me to die than to live." And the LORD said, "Do you do well to be angry?"*

Jonah went out of the city and sat to the east of the city and made a booth for himself there. He sat under it in the shade, till he should see what would become of the city. **Now** *the* LORD *God appointed a plant and made it come up over Jonah, that it might be a shade over his head, to save him from his discomfort. So Jonah was exceedingly glad because of the plant. But when dawn came up the next day, God appointed a worm that attacked the plant, so that it withered. When the sun rose, God appointed a scorching east wind, and the sun beat down on the head of Jonah so that he was faint. And he asked that he might die and said, "It is better for me to die than to live." But God said to Jonah, "Do you do well to be angry for the plant?" And he said, "Yes, I do well to be angry, angry enough to die." And the* LORD *said, "You pity the plant, for which you did not labor, nor did you make it grow, which came into being in a night and perished in a night. And should not I pity Nineveh, that great city, in which there are more than 120,000 persons who do not know their right hand from their left, and also much cattle?"(Jonah 3:6–Micah)*

This is the attitude God *doesn't* want us to have: hatred, anger, condemnation, and unforgiveness. Have you ever felt this way about someone? Wanting them to suffer and perish? Jesus said to those who did the harm to Him that He forgave them and asked His Father to do the same. His love moved Him to do so. That is the face and identity of genuine *Unlossable Love.* We are commanded to share this same love. It's not just a suggestion…

UNLOSSABLE LOVE TOWARDS OURSELVES

Are we revisiting this again? Didn't we already cover this? Yes, and no. We have touched on this, but not to the extent to which we need to. I also know from personal experience that we often revisit it from time to time because we continue to hold ourselves to a different level of accountability than we do our loved ones or even strangers. Why is that? Does this happen to you?

People can be forgiven and offered *Unlossable Love* for various reasons which we have covered in earlier chapters. To forgive ourselves and to offer that love to me? That's a very different story. It's easy to extend this to others because we have an already established love or relationship with that person, we have limited knowledge of the entire person and choose to not see their flaws, we might be trained by our faith systems/religion, or even by our upbringing in the family systems we were a part of. With these, we can choose to ignore certain aspects, "see what we want to see and believe what we want to believe" or be influenced by others. We can escape at any time and isolate different unpleasant thoughts and feelings by detaching ourselves from situations and circumstances. Some professional counselors call this *compartmentalization*—having the ability to place thoughts and feelings into a tidy compartment in our mind or heart and lock it away until we decide to address it; if we ever decide to address it, that is.

I became a master of this because of the different professions/callings God has called me to as both a pastor and a mental health professional.

Unlossable Love Towards Ourselves

In working with individuals that come from a wide variety of situations and circumstances (some of which they created by the poor choices they have made, while other circumstances were thrust upon them by individuals), I walked with some of these families and individuals in some of their deepest and darkest moments. Some of the experiences were so horrific that they became newsworthy. Several times I had to appear in court to testify about some of those circumstances.

In being a pastor, much like that being in the mental health field, you are held to confidentiality. This being said, one can only begin to imagine all of the various emotions and feelings that a person can feel as they help others go through their struggles and having no outlet except through God to be able to deal with your own thoughts and feelings, your re-traumatization and your own self-doubt about if you have what it takes to help these individuals through their circumstances.

I had learned to de-compartmentalize thoughts and feelings and to tuck them away into neat little corners of my soul. Like a computer, I was able to go back and forth into these little files in my heart as needed and keep them organized the best way I saw fit. And just like a computer, I discovered that some of those files had "viruses" (negative effects that one never realized this is infiltrating your hard drive until it's too late) that had affected me more deeply than I ever imagined.

Upon discovering this, I began to do some soul-searching to see how this impacted me. When I look at various ways in which those that I tried to help have traumatized me, I understood that the reason for this taking place was because I had never fully dealt with some of the situations in my own past. When you tuck things away, you often forget about these things. I understood that when you tuck things away, there always is a day of reckoning. As that day approaches, and you never know when that day is, when you store things away, it catches us off guard and compounds are situations far greater than if we would have dealt with them at that present time of experiencing it firsthand. You sometimes discover that you are doing the exact same things, but you are teaching others not to do or to avoid doing. You lie to yourself and say that it is not hypocritical; justifying it by saying that you are addressing the issues at your own pace. Then God challenges you to be honest with yourself and your guilt begins to thicken and compound itself more and more in your soul.

Shortly after this revelation, I began to follow the leadership of the Holy Spirit and practice some of the evidence-based practices that I was teaching others and how to deal with the various issues I personally had. As I began to model those things that I understood were from God and use the application of the various tools and skills that I possess, I began to realize that my ability to love not only others, but myself, strengthened. As I became involved in accountability groups (an accountability group is a group of people that you hand-select to become your most intimate of relationships and you place total trust in, in which all or part of this group be vulnerable with one another, who brutally be honest with you about your choices and actions and will hold you accountable to the things that you commit to; and you do the same for them), I learned to address my past and present history. During the process, I discovered that as I unpacked my baggage, I was able to find my ability to receive *Unlossable Love* for myself and truly mean it! The more I was exposed to this love, my self-worth improved, and I became a more effective pastor and mental health worker. I was able to "delete" the need for emotional and mental storage bins; thus, freeing me in ways that I never knew I needed. My relationships improved, my self-esteem and confidence returned, and I could begin to see improvements in those I serve.

Because of seeing and experiencing God's agape/*Unlossable Love*, I was able to see the possibility of allowing myself the healing from it and learned how to love myself; not in an arrogant manner, but in a way that would transform me and heal my poor opinion of myself. I will admit that there are/will be times when I might try to slip back into old habits and isolation; lowering my ability to love and forgive myself. After all, I am human. Now, with the help of my accountability brothers, I can avoid going back and am able to keep moving forward.

Let me ask you a question: what obstacles are preventing you from granting permission for you to allow yourself the healing of *Unlossable Love* for yourself and to yourself? In my account, I realized the baggage I carried hindered my healing and interfered with more than I considered. As you search for your own life, please be honest with yourself. It is the only way you can finally put to rest the past and begin to see your worth to God and the world around you. If you are not honest with yourself as you do this self-examination of your soul and spirit, you will not find the answers that you seek and you will forever remain stuck where you are. It is extremely important in your self-examination to unlock and unpack all those boxes that you have hidden in your mind and your heart. If this means you need the assistance of close friends and family to help you unpack, make sure that those individuals are the same individuals who will be honest with you and love you at the same time. Judgment will only cause you to lock those things away all the deeper and to place more locks to make them impenetrable by not only others but yourself.

Another wise thing to apply here is God's love toward us in all manners of His love. If you are not a person of faith, this is where you might consider having a relationship with God. Because God is love and the author of *Unlossable Love*, who better to learn from than the author Himself? I guide you to the relationship with God because of the difference that my relationship with God has transformed my life. From personal experience, I went from having no self-esteem and no value (as I could see and perceive it) to becoming an individual who is able to see the valuable gift that God made me to be and to mirror His love towards myself and others. I share God because I love him so dearly and I share God because I love you so dearly. It is because of you, the readers, that I write what God puts on my heart so that you may be able to hear (possibly for the first time), how God sees you and values you. If you are the only one who had ever lived, God would have still sent Jesus just for you so that you may have salvation in peace in His agape/*Unlossable Love*. God longs to have an intimate relationship with you.

As you begin your self-examination, you will discover that you tucked away more than you ever imagined, and this might overwhelm you. Just like if you are to move from one physical home to another; you discover that you have more things than you realize. When this happens, is up to you to decide what to unpack first (the most important to deal with) and then the order after that.

I had just recently moved from a church community in which I was their pastor for 21 years, and then God called me to my current church community. We had to pack up everything into moving trucks. As we were packing up boxes of those things that we use most often, we discovered that we had many boxes that were already packed and had not seen the light of day for years. We still had to take those boxes with us to our new home.

Once we got everything into our new home, and we had all the boxes all over the place, we began to unpack. We had to prioritize which items we needed right now and unpacked those first. Once we got the necessities taken care of, we began to unpack those items that were bulky we put them in the proper places where they needed to go. By doing this, we were able to de-clutter a great deal of the space that they took when they were in storage.

We did not rush through the unpacking and we took our time to truly evaluate those things that we wanted to keep and use, those things that we wanted to keep but store (because we realize that we would need these in the near future and that these items are used on sporadic moments), and those things that we realized were things that we kept

Unlossable Love Towards Ourselves

that either had no meaning to us or that interfered with our home. We left those things in boxes and removed them from our lives by giving them to donation centers or we simply threw them away. The more that we de-cluttered, the more beautiful and inviting our home became and our pride in our home increased. We were also able to realize the rest and peace that we were able to experience moving forward because we realized that once we were done unpacking, it was finally over.

This is the type of approach that you must follow for yourself. You must realize all that you have stored within your heart and soul into considering what you need to purge from your life. You must base it upon your own decision on what you must unpack first and the importance of this and focus on that alone. Only after you have completely unpacked that, you move on to the next box, then the next box, and so on.

As you get the assistance of others who have helped to move to this point, don't allow them to dictate to you what is needed first; you are alone with the choice of what to unpack first and where to place it. I say this because you are the one who is going to live with yourself every day in these other individuals, even though they may be significant parts of your life, they may not fully understand your rhyme and reason for doing the things that you do the way that you do. And if you utilize the magnifying glass of *Unlossable Love*, you'll see clearly how this will help maneuver you through the deepest troubles of your life and finally put to rest those things that should have been laid to rest so long ago.

The one thing that we discovered in our move and when the moving trucks had placed all of the boxes and personal belongings into the home, we discovered that we had no room to move around: we cannot move our furniture to where we wanted it to be, we were unable to get to our cooking utensils or our bedding for other things that we needed for the day to day things. This is where we had to prioritize and search for those most needed items. Our very basic need in life is love: to love and to be loved. When love is absent, we believe ourselves to have no value and no purpose in life. Even though that statement makes sense, it becomes a very dangerous position to hold on to because we limit our value. As shared throughout the book, God's agape/*Unlossable Love* is never removed or taken away, but it can be placed behind the veil of our own irrational thought processes, misconceptions taught to us through generational experiences, or the lies that we choose to believe in that others tried to make our reality. Knowing how God loves us and empowers us to be able to see, even with blurred eyes, enables us to behold the possibilities that lie within each of us through that love.

Having the ability to allow ourselves to love and forgive ourselves is as important as your next breath: if you're not able to breathe deep that life-giving breath, you will die. If you can't accept love from yourself, how do you expect to give love to others? You can't give what you do not have. When we discussed the various types of love, which one can you offer? To offer a superficial form of love to a person who needs the agape love of God and/or *Unlossable Love*, can produce a situation with irreparable damages; if that individual has been looking for true love and acceptance and we offer them the same type of shallow love or false love, we can actually push them over the edge to the point where they will refuse to accept any sort of love whatsoever. (I shared my personal experience with this earlier in the book.) If it wasn't for God and those who had intervened on my behalf, God only knows where I would be today.

Hopefully, you're beginning to see the importance of having the ability to have *Unlossable Love* for yourself to be able to make the necessary changes that you desire within yourself. Let this love motivate you to know your true worth that is not based on acts of work or on the opinion of others. You deserve love for yourself. Let it help you to take proper care of yourself in every aspect of your life You will soon discover how it will make more room within your heart for God and others; without tripping over yourself.

BIBLICAL EXAMPLES OF GOD'S UNLOSSABLE LOVE

In my mind, I had pondered if there were any biblical examples that I could share to show how long God's agape/*Unlossable Love* has been involved in man's life. I thought to myself, "*Who was the first person to receive God's Unlossable Love?*" I prayed and studied this and of course, God shows up in a BIG way! God took me back to the beginning when Adam and Eve fell from grace.

> *And they heard the sound of the* Lord *God walking in the garden in the cool of the day, and the man and his wife hid themselves from the presence of the* Lord *God among the trees of the garden. But the* Lord *God called to the man and said to him, "Where are you?" And he said, "I heard the sound of you in the garden, and I was afraid, because I was naked, and I hid myself." He said, "Who told you that you were naked? Have you eaten of the tree of which I commanded you not to eat?" The man said, "The woman whom you gave to be with me, she gave me fruit of the tree, and I ate." Then the* Lord *God said to the woman, "What is this that you have done?" The woman said, "The serpent deceived me, and I ate."*
>
> *The* Lord *God said to the serpent,*
> *"Because you have done this, cursed are you above all livestock and above all beasts of the field;*

*on your belly you shall go,
and dust you shall eat
all the days of your life.
I will put enmity between you and the woman,
and between your offspring and her offspring;
he shall bruise your head,
and you shall bruise his heel."
To the woman he said,
"I will surely multiply your pain in childbearing;
in pain you shall bring forth children.
Your desire shall be contrary to your husband,
but he shall rule over you."
And to Adam he said,
"Because you have listened to the voice of your wife
and have eaten of the tree
of which I commanded you,
'You shall not eat of it,'
cursed is the ground because of you;
in pain you shall eat of it all the days of your life;
thorns and thistles it shall bring forth for you;
and you shall eat the plants of the field.
By the sweat of your face
you shall eat bread,
till you return to the ground,
for out of it you were taken;
for you are dust,
and to dust you shall return."
    The man called his wife's name Eve, because she was the mother of all living. And the* L<small>ORD</small> *God made for Adam and for his wife garments of skins and clothed them. (Genesis 3:8–21)*

Biblical Examples of God's Unlossable Love

After reading this, you might be saying, "Seriously? Where does he see God's agape/*Unlossable Love* evident here? Believe me, it's here in this passage. Let's investigate . . .

If you are familiar with this biblical text, Satan, disguised as the serpent, seduces and abuses God's creation of man. Satan knew the best way to get even with God for expelling him from Heaven was to corrupt and destroy the relationship between God and man. The woman (Eve) is taken advantage of by the serpent, and he tricks her to disobey what God had told Adam. When the Fall takes place and Eve shares with God the details, God delivers justice to the serpent. (As you read the rest of the Bible, you'll discover that Satan's justice is ongoing from when he was cast out of Heaven until when Christ returns.)

As for Adam and Eve, God's *Unlossable Love* is noted by His walk with them daily in the Garden. Yes, it was before the Fall, yet it shows God's desire for connectedness with His creation and especially man. After the Fall from grace, God continued to love and care for man allowing the natural consequence to be invoked. *What? How is that Unlossable Love?* First, God was not a liar; He informed man what would happen, and it did: man chose sin over obedience and their relationship, and its purity died at that moment. God's *Unlossable Love* allows man to experience the consequences of his actions to show him what He (God) was trying to prevent in the first place.

A good modern example is how we, as parents, tell our young children to not reach up on a hot stove; our love is trying to prevent the children from great pain and suffering. If the child disobeys our instructions, they face the natural (and painful) consequences of their actions. The loving parents don't leave them in their suffering but attend to the wounds and attempt to bring healing and restoration to the children. God does this with us and for us.

Next, we see God clothing Adam and Eve. This meant a sacrifice might have needed to be made; although it is unclear if one was made.

It is certain that because of the Fall, there had to be a covering for the sinful act. Prior to the Fall, Adam and Eve were innocent of wrongdoing. They fellowshipped with God. After the Fall, a holy God could not be in the presence of sin without a covering for man and God provided such a covering so fellowship would continue. This covering also serves as a reminder to man that for man to have ongoing intimacy with God, his shame must be addressed. God provides adequate clothing for Adam and Eve. Once again, God's love steps in to keep the relationship with man open.

Following the Fall, Adam and Eve conceive, and she gives birth to Cain. Take note of what Eve declares: *"Now Adam knew Eve his wife, and she conceived and bore Cain, saying, "I have gotten a man with the help of the LORD." (Genesis 4:1)*

"With the help of the LORD." This is evidence that God continued to be involved with a man and does what He can to preserve and restore man unto Himself. As Able was born and matured, we see stark differences between Cain and Able. Able seeks to serve God and is obedient; while Cain followed the same path which his parents had walked and didn't follow the leadership of God. Cain was upset because Abel's offerings were acceptable and he wasn't. Read on . . .

> *And the LORD had regard for Abel and his offering, but for Cain and his offering he had no regard. So Cain was very angry, and his face fell. The LORD said to Cain, "Why are you angry, and why has your face fallen? If you do well, will you not be accepted? And if you do not do well, sin is crouching at the door. Its desire is contrary to you, but you must rule over it."(Genesis 4:4–7)*

God is open and honest; explaining what must be done for his offerings to be accepted. God also addresses Cain's anger problems. Does Cain accept the help and guidance? Is he willing to be obedient?

No. Cain has Able to take a walk with him and then kills Able. What is God's response to this?

> *Cain spoke to Abel his brother. And when they were in the field, Cain rose up against his brother Abel and killed him. Then the LORD said to Cain, "Where is Abel your brother?" He said, "I do not know; am I my brother's keeper?" And the LORD said, "What have you done? The voice of your brother's blood is crying to me from the ground. And now you are cursed from the ground, which has opened its mouth to receive your brother's blood from your hand. When you work the ground, it shall no longer yield to you its strength. You shall be a fugitive and a wanderer on the earth." Cain said to the LORD, "My punishment is greater than I can bear. Behold, you have driven me today away from the ground, and from your face I shall be hidden. I shall be a fugitive and a wanderer on the earth, and whoever finds me will kill me." Then the LORD said to him, "Not so! If anyone kills Cain, vengeance shall be taken on him sevenfold." And the LORD put a mark on Cain, lest any who found him should attack him. Then Cain went away from the presence of the LORD and settled in the land of Nod, east of Eden. (Genesis 4:8–16)*

With Abel's death, as we look through man's eyes, Cain deserved the same fate. Man's sin once again is exposed to God. Does God deal with Cain as he deserves? No. Once again, God's agape/*Unlossable Love* intervenes and provides mercy. Man's mercy is shown in Cain's acts against his brother, while God's acts continue to offer redemption for man. This goes on throughout the Scriptures and into today's generations to today's people. This same love of God isn't based on what we do or don't do but is *Unlossable Love*. People place conditions on whom they love, how they love, and what warrants the removal of that love. God's love has no such conditions, it simply is ever-present.

Another example of this is David. Most of us know the story of how he took on a giant named Goliath. That was just the beginning of his story. (To see the entire story, read both 1 and 2 Samuel and the first two chapters of 1 Kings.) David did many great things, and at the same time, equally poor things. In the end, David is regarded as a man after God's own heart. David had natural consequences for his actions of adultery, murder, and so on. The reason why God still considered David and others (Abraham, Moses, Sampson, Solomon to name a few) as men after His own heart is because they took ownership of their mistakes and poor choices, did what was required, and served the consequences, repented, and re-established their relationship with God. Remember what God told Cain? These men took God's advice and turned things around.

Unlossable Love doesn't give permission to do wrong or to sin; it provides a way for us to be restored and to follow the advice that God gave Cain. You can see that every one of our biblical heroes and heroines, had moments of poor choices, mistakes, and outright sin between the miracles God did through them. The only time these choices discounted them from grace is when they chose to continue in their choices to be apart from God (Judas, Saul from David's story in the Samuel books, the Rich Ruler from the Luke 18 passage, and more are examples of this). God's love never stopped or lessened a single ounce.

As we search the Scriptures, we can see the most amazing displays of God's love put to work through Jesus Christ. Jesus would be approached by numerous people who desired healing, restoration, and forgiveness. His love would address the needs, point out the sin and/or sinful habits and attitudes, give us directions to stop the sinning or wrongful actions, and restore the relationships that desired to be resurrected.

What does this do for us today? As in the days of the Scriptures, the same God gives us the same opportunities for forgiveness, restoration, and intimacy that He had with those whom Scripture records. God's love never changes, His approaches haven't changed, and His desire for intimacy remains a constant for today's generations.

DEVELOPING OUR ACCESSIBILITY TO UNLOSSABLE LOVE

It's been great to discuss *Unlossable Love* from God and what it means to us; but how do *we* develop *our accessibility* to *Unlossable Love* for mankind? There are plenty of factors to consider in such a task. In our discussions prior to this chapter, we must first understand what exactly this love is. This is a new term that this book hopefully explains to all.

The understanding of *Unlossable Love* develops the desire for it in our lives. When Beatrice shared her testimony, she discovered what it meant to her without knowing exactly what it was until years later. She experienced that which she couldn't identify. Have you ever tried to express a feeling that you couldn't pinpoint? To our frustrations, when we don't have an identity, we can't appropriately share our thoughts and feelings to where we are understood. Beatrice was able to share with her family that love because she was exposed to the *Unlossable Love* we now write about.

We also shared about the origins of this love being God. He created this love and IS this love. We now have an example from which we can draw to recreate this love in our daily lives and with those we love. We spoke briefly about how to acquire *Unlossable Love* from one another; now, let's get down to details. . . .

As I was growing up, there was a man named Richard "Rich" Little. In my youth, I wanted to be just like him because he did many different voice impersonations. I thought to myself, "How cool is that! I want to learn how to do that!" I mean, he was spot-on in his impersonations and I wondered how he did it.

I watched Rich in an interview with I believe (but can't say for certain because that was in my youth, and I am FAR removed from that youth…) David Frost and David asked how long it takes him (Rich) to learn a new voice. Rich had informed David that it depends on the person's tone, voice patterns, and mannerisms. Rich went on to say that he had to listen to the person for a great deal of time and to practice their voice multiple times. Some, Rich explained, came easy because his real voice was close to their voices. For others, it took months of practice to master. Even after mastering this skill, Rich had to continually practice their voice to *maintain the ability* to keep that voice.

Likewise, we are to do the very same with *Unlossable Love* if we are to use it to its fullest potential. The word Unlossable means it doesn't stop and that it continues. As a parent loves their children, they continually present that love in every aspect of the child's/children's life. A husband and wife should be sharing this every day of their lives. Siblings are also required to maintain this standard of love.

Now, to address those who are unfamiliar with *Unlossable Love*: How do we gain access to this love? After identifying this love, we need to develop a desire for it. That desire drives us to obtain it.

Going back to the Rich Little example; being exposed to his talents caused me to desire the development of that same talent for myself. Throughout the years and being exposed to the talents of Robin Williams and others, I learned how to also impersonate different celebrities and artists. Granted, I am *nowhere* near the talent that these guys were, but I can make several impressions and can do them well. It did take a great deal of practice and once acquired; I continually practice keeping that ability up to the standard to which I have grown accustomed. Likewise, it is important for us to familiarize ourselves with *Unlossable Love* and to practice it with those that we love and with ourselves.

If we want to build up muscle mass and be toned, we must put in the effort to build those muscles that we want to focus on. We cannot start out by trying to lift 300 pounds at one time when we have never done that before. We must examine ourselves to see what our limitations are and to discover how to best work up our endurance to be able to obtain the maximum weight that our bodies can lift. Then we must do the work of putting in the hours, the sweat, and the effort to be able to meet that goal that we have achieved. Some will progress quickly, while others might take a bit more time to develop. Either way, the goals can be met if we are devoted to the cause.

Man is conditioned to expect results after they try something out instead of before trying it out. Commercials are perfect examples of this truth. When a product wants you to purchase it, they convince you, the viewer, that it's something *you can't live without*! They compare their product to others like it and show you that *my product* is far superior to the competition's product. They show you the difference between each; *but wait, there's more!!!* . . . Next, they have "actual users" of said product and they give testimony to how their lives have now been completed because of said product. "But wait! There's more. . . act right now and we'll include . . . " is always the next to last line; placing urgency on your accepting their pitch and getting you to commit to their product. Maybe they'll double the product or add another item you can't live without. The icing on the cake is that they will add free shipping *if you act RIGHT NOW*! So, then we send our money to them, and get our products; only to discover that the promises they made didn't live up to our expectations. Why did I add this illustration? It serves the purpose of understanding that we can be taken advantage of if we let our guard down.

I shared that illustration of weightlifting and muscle development to express the need to assess our goals and desires and to carefully examine not just the goal, but the method to said goal. The commercial example shows how even in relationships, we are pressured into some relationships that promise to make our lives complete; only to take advantage of us. Many of us have experienced a relationship like this or have witnessed it in the life of someone we love. They deplete us of our emotional bank accounts, making us mentally, emotionally, and even spiritually bankrupt.

To know how to access *Unlossable Love*, we need to know what it can do for us. Beatrice was able to share this love with her family and foster children *because she had a clear understanding of what Unlossable Love was* (as stated in her earlier testimony), *saw the impact on her life, and then shared it with those she loves.* She knew the Author of that love (God), who is a trusted source (I dare say the most trusted source), she put it to the test and discovered the Promises of God are real. She integrated this love in her life towards others and herself and the end results are everything and more than she expected. What made the difference? *Application.*

The application of *Unlossable Love* first begins with us. God has shown us this love in this way:

> *Therefore, since we have been justified by faith, we have peace with God through our Lord Jesus Christ. Through him we have also obtained access by faith into this grace in which we stand, and we rejoice in hope of the glory of God. Not only that, but we rejoice in our sufferings, knowing that suffering produces endurance, and endurance produces character, and character produces hope, and hope does not put us to shame, because God's love has been poured into our hearts through the Holy Spirit who has been given to us.*
>
> *For while we were still weak, at the right time Christ died for the ungodly. For one will scarcely die for a righteous person—though perhaps for a good person one would dare even to die—* **but** *God shows his love for us in that while we were still sinners, Christ died*

> *for us. Since, therefore, we have now been justified by his blood, much more shall we be saved by him from the wrath of God. For if while we were enemies we were reconciled to God by the death of his Son, much more, now that we are reconciled, shall we be saved by his life. More than that, we also rejoice in God through our Lord Jesus Christ, through whom we have now received reconciliation. (Romans 5:1–11)*

Dying for the ungodly, the sinner, for all. While we were *enemies*; this is a powerful statement because it means we are at odds with one another in conflict. And yet, He still loves us with His agape/*Unlossable Love*! The application of our faith in God allows us to accept His love and then we apply it to our lives. Once the application of His love is within us, its healing power begins to work its miracles and not only heals us but transforms us in the understanding that THIS is the love we have always been searching for! We become living testimonies of God's love because of God's love.

A biblical example of this is found in the book of John in the Scriptures. It involves Jesus and a woman at a well. As you read this passage, please note the effects of Jesus' love and compassion for this woman and the impact of this love on herself and others:

> *Now when Jesus learned that the Pharisees had heard that Jesus was making and baptizing more disciples than John (although Jesus himself did not baptize, but only his disciples), he left Judea and departed again for Galilee. And he had to pass through Samaria. So he came to a town of Samaria called Sychar, near the field that Jacob had given to his son Joseph. Jacob's well was there; so Jesus, wearied as he was from his journey, was sitting beside the well. It was about the sixth hour.*
>
> *A woman from Samaria came to draw water. Jesus said to her, "Give me a drink." (For his disciples had gone away into the city to*

buy food.) The Samaritan woman said to him, "How is it that you, a Jew, ask for a drink from me, a woman of Samaria?" (For Jews have no dealings with Samaritans.) Jesus answered her, "If you knew the gift of God, and who it is that is saying to you, 'Give me a drink,' you would have asked him, and he would have given you living water." The woman said to him, "Sir, you have nothing to draw water with, and the well is deep. Where do you get that living water? Are you greater than our father Jacob? He gave us the well and drank from it himself, as did his sons and his livestock." Jesus said to her, "Everyone who drinks of this water will be thirsty again, but whoever drinks of the water that I will give him will never be thirsty again. The water that I will give him will become in him a spring of water welling up to eternal life." The woman said to him, "Sir, give me this water, so that I will not be thirsty or have to come here to draw water."

Jesus said to her, "Go, call your husband, and come here." The woman answered him, "I have no husband." Jesus said to her, "You are right in saying, 'I have no husband'; for you have had five husbands, and the one you now have is not your husband. What you have said is true." The woman said to him, "Sir, I perceive that you are a prophet. Our fathers worshiped on this mountain, but you say that in Jerusalem is the place where people ought to worship." Jesus said to her, "Woman, believe me, the hour is coming when neither on this mountain nor in Jerusalem will you worship the Father. You worship what you do not know; we worship what we know, for salvation is from the Jews. But the hour is coming, and is now here, when the true worshipers will worship the Father in spirit and truth, for the Father is seeking such people to worship him. **God** is spirit, and those who worship him must worship in spirit and truth." The woman said to him, "I know that Messiah is coming (he who is called Christ). When he comes, he will tell us all things." Jesus said to her, "I who speak to you am he."

> *Just then his disciples came back. They marveled that he was talking with a woman, but no one said, "What do you seek?" or, "Why are you talking with her?" So the woman left her water jar and went away into town and said to the people, "Come, see a man who told me all that I ever did. Can this be the Christ?" They went out of the town and were coming to him.*
>
> *Meanwhile the disciples were urging him, saying, "Rabbi, eat." But he said to them, "I have food to eat that you do not know about." So the disciples said to one another, "Has anyone brought him something to eat?" Jesus said to them, "My food is to do the will of him who sent me and to accomplish his work. Do you not say, 'There are yet four months, then comes the harvest'? Look, I tell you, lift up your eyes, and see that the fields are ripe for harvest. Already the one who reaps is receiving wages and gathering fruit for eternal life, so that sower and reaper may rejoice together. For here the saying holds true, 'One sows and another reaps.' I sent you to reap that for which you did not labor. Others have labored, and you have entered into their labor."*
>
> *Many Samaritans from that town believed in him because of the woman's testimony, "He told me all that I ever did." So when the Samaritans came to him, they asked him to stay with them, and he stayed there two days. And many more believed because of his word. They said to the woman, "It is no longer because of what you said that we believe, for we have heard for ourselves, and we know that this is indeed the Savior of the world." (John 4:1–42)*

Jesus met this woman at Jacob's well. She was a Samaritan, from an outcast group of people who combined the Jewish religion and pagan faiths into one belief system—thus desecrating themselves from what God had called the Jewish people to be set apart from other faiths to be the example God called them to be. Jesus wasn't supposed to be even in their land; let alone be talking to "such people". Add the fact that with her being a woman and the custom of that time was that a man shouldn't be talking with a woman of her reputation to avoid suspicion, and Jesus had gone *way* outside the box (norm) to present the love of His Father to someone who had little or no self-value because of not only poor choices but social norms of that day.

Jesus established communication and trust with this woman, proved that He knew her intimately in a non-judgmental way (explaining to her about not only her past, but her current situation in such a way that she wasn't looked down upon, but He was actually lifting her up), introduced her to God's love and forgiveness and applied that love to her heart. That love became the Living Water and flowed within her soul; transforming her to become a conduit for God's agape/*Unlossable Love* to flow from her to her community. This caused the people from her town to come and see this love at work for themselves. They too experienced this love, and they accredit her for this transformation because she was not only transformed, but also shared that love with others. That is an example of what such love can do if we expose ourselves to this love, accept and apply it and then share it with others. One person (Jesus) met one person's needs (the woman), she accepted and applied that healing love, was transformed and healed, and then testified to the saving grace of God.

In the same manner, as Jesus developed God's love within the woman at the well, she, in turn, developed it within others. She witnessed this love in Christ and saw the need for this love to be present in her life. She then embraces that love that was restored to her, and then shared it with her city. Today, we have the humble privilege and honor to have the same effect as this woman at the well. If we follow the leadership of the Holy Spirit that sometimes calls us to break norms and to reach out in love and compassion, we too can experience not only the healing touch for ourselves; we just might be able to impact the world around us. Our accessibility to the Author (God) and to those who possess *Unlossable Love* empowers us to have this capability to do the same.

CAUSE AND EFFECT OF UNLOSSABLE LOVE

You might be asking yourself, "Why would he put in a chapter about '. . . cause and effect' for *Unlossable Love*? As we just noted in the last chapter, love is not only actional but also *reactional*. The effects of a town responding to a sinful woman's transformation came directly from her encounter with Jesus (the cause). This illustration is powerful because all parties involved were ready for it to take place. The conditions were right at the right time. What might have happened if even *one thing* was different? Would the outcome be different? ABSOLUTELY!! Let's investigate . . . using the same passage from John...

Timing—What if the timing was off? What if Jesus appeared at the well at a different time of the day? In the passage, it was important to disclose the time of day. (We will address a possible reason for it shortly.) *"It was midday. The Jewish day runs from 6 a.m. to 6 p.m. and the sixth hour is twelve o'clock midday. So the heat was at its greatest, and Jesus was weary and thirsty from traveling.* [5]*"*

The significance of the timing shows the time of day was when most people wouldn't come to the well because it was the hottest time of the day. Most would have drawn water earlier in the day or later when it began to cool down. If Jesus would have come at a different time, Jesus would have met someone else, and the story would be different.

---

5 Barclay, William, ed., (1975). *The Gospel of John* (Vol. 1, p. 147). (Louisville, Ken.: Westminster John Knox Press, 1975), 147.

Unlossable Love

The same can be said for the woman's timing. She could have possibly not had an encounter with the Living Water.

Reason for coming to the well—without the simple understanding of why Jesus stopped by the well (He was tired and thirsty), the focus turns towards the woman: what reason did she feel the need to come to the well at the time she did? *"As Jesus sat there, there came to the well a Samaritan woman. Why she should come to that well is something of a mystery, for it was more than half-a-mile from Sychar where she must have stayed and there was water there. May it be that she was so much of a moral outcast that the women even drove her away from the village well and she had to come here to draw water?* [6]*"*

In several different commentaries, it is noted that this woman's reputation was most likely the cause of her coming to the well at that time of day. Whether it was her choice to go at that time because of the inner shame she placed upon herself, social pressure and shame that took place, or a combination of both, she was compelled to draw water at that time and at this well. If the woman had gone to a different well or water source, again, the meeting probably wouldn't have taken place.

Customs—religious and social customs should have prevented the encounter. John the Beloved (Jesus' Disciple and writer of the Gospel of John) shares in the passage the social distance each should have kept from one another. Even just speaking to such a woman with her background could have caused great controversy for Jesus and His reputation. Religious leaders wouldn't engage with such a woman alone to avoid the gossip and drama which could and often arise in doing so.

> *Jesus asked her to give him a drink. She turned in astonishment. "I am a Samaritan," she said. "You are a Jew. How is it that you ask a drink from me?" And then John explains to the Greeks*

---

6 Barclay, *The Gospel of John*, p. 148

for whom he is writing that there was no kind of come and go at all between the Jews and the Samaritans.

Now it is certain that all we have here is the briefest possible report of what must have been a long conversation. Clearly there was much more to this meeting than is recorded here. If we may use an analogy, this is like the minutes of a committee meeting where we have only the salient points of the discussion recorded. I think that the Samaritan woman must have unburdened her soul to this stranger. How else could Jesus have known of her tangled domestic affairs? For one of the very few times in her life she had found one with kindness in his eyes instead of critical superiority; and she opened her heart.

Few stories in the Gospel record show us so much about the character of Jesus.[7]

Barclay's commentary gives some proper insight into what probably transpired between Jesus and this woman. If the Disciples went to the town of Sychar for food, this was at least half a mile from the well. Add the time to find the food and to return to where Jesus was, it is reasonable to say that Jesus and this woman could have talked for at least an hour or two together. Barclay asks the question about how Jesus might have known about this woman's "tangled domestic affairs." I would suggest that Jesus, being very much man and very much God, knows all. John also indicates this in his recount by the way he writes this account and that it is Jesus which points these truths out to the woman; which in turn causes the woman to declare Jesus as a prophet.

The account of this woman's interaction with Jesus had to have happened as John records it to have the only outcome that it did. Numerous choices were made and the reactions to those choices produced

---

7 Barclay, *The Gospel of John*, p. 148.

the effective outcome God desired for not only the woman but her entire town as well.

What causes us to desire to change, to love, to remain where we are or to move on, or to do whatever we desire to do? Comfort or lack of comfort, contentment or lack of contentment, peace or chaos, and happiness or emptiness are a few of the many reasons for a change. Sometimes, these are well thought out and other times come from impulsive actions. Everything we do is a choice that carries an action and reaction or response. There is no escaping it; there's a cause and effect to every choice we have. If I choose to not look at the weather forecast and just go out into the day without that information, I go unprepared for what the elements hold. I could experience being too hot or cold, exposed to too much sun or in need of an umbrella, walking into a tornado, or strolling in the fog; all because my choice was to not look at the forecast.

It is not limited to just our choices, but also the choices of others which also have even deeper causes and effects. No child ever desires to go into the foster care system; the actions and choices of others (or sometimes their actions/choices) cause them to be removed from their biological family's home. Abuse, neglect, trauma, loss of income, loss of a family member due to death/divorce/separation, and health issues which the individual has no control over also have causes and effects; especially how *we respond to* the situation(s). These also have an impact on things, and they continually go back and forth, and we dance this way all our lives.

Does this mean we have no control or choice? We can influence the causes and effects with our responses. If we choose God's agape/ *Unlossable Love* to be in our lives, the outcome produces positive and desired reactions. Should we choose anger and bitterness to our circumstances, the reactions will most likely be equally as negative as our response (I say most likely because if God has allowed the other person's response or choice to influence our actions, God might be using *them* to reach *us*). We might not have full control of what happens to us; however, we have *total* control over our responses to our actions.

Recall for me, if you will, the last argument you were engaged in: what was it like? What was it about? What happened during the disagreement? How did the other person(s) respond to you? How long did it last? What happened at the end? Was it ended peacefully or is it still ongoing? I asked you to recall this to see if my cause and effect is spot on or if I missed the mark. Let me give you this probable response and see how well I do:

Someone did or said something to you that created a negative response or feeling within you. Your reaction was to address the incident with the other individual(s) by reacting to the same level of negativity (or you might have even kicked it up a notch). The talking gets faster and higher. You both are wanting to be heard, but the other isn't listening. As the argument becomes more intense, the talking becomes yelling, and tempers continue to rise. Each of you now is saying things without regard to the other's feelings and emotions are out of control. This continues back and forth between one another until someone else "who is in control" of themselves attempts to calm the situation down, someone tries to turn it physical, someone leaves or something is able to bring you back to being civil with one another and talking resumes.

Was I on point or way off? Why would you say this? *Choices you made.* How you responded was a choice. Their response was a choice. To escalate or de-escalate was a choice. To stay or leave, to listen to the others trying to defuse the fight, and the decision to get physical or resume talking are all choices. The scenario changes with each response and decision. Depending on what you did dictates the result. You can cause the effect you desire by modeling that same response.

In my training for the mental health field and in working with troubled youth, we were trained on how to de-escalate volatile situations.

If the other person is yelling, acting out verbally, and possibly physically aggressively, we are called to keep a soft voice as much as possible and to show calmness. Any hint of agitation from us would and often did escalate the situation. The more we remained calm, the quicker the situation was resolved, and the less damage physically, mentally, and emotionally occurred to all involved.

Love is that calmness and the changing agent which will bring peace to the situations we engage in. Love produces respect, respect produces trust, and trust produces obedience. God's love produces a calmness that allows respect to be shared with all parties. When we respect someone, even in conflict, trust becomes apparent because they see we are not trying to hurt them or dishonor them. That builds trust that allows rational thoughts to be shared, heard, and reflected on one another. Trust shows respect, which finally leads to resolutions that are positive for all involved.

If a person understands and has *Unlossable Love* granted to them, this causes a foundation of value for the person receiving it. It is a strong, solid foundation that can weather any storm that is thrown at it. Jesus had a great deal to share about having a firm foundation:

> *Everyone who comes to me and hears my words and does them, I will show you what he is like:* **he is** *like a man building a house, who dug deep and laid the foundation on the rock. And when a flood arose, the stream broke against that house and could not shake it, because it had been well built. But the one who hears and does not do them is like a man who built a house on the ground without a foundation. When the stream broke against it, immediately it fell, and the ruin of that house was great. (Luke 6:47-49)*

I share this with you because just like in our faith in God, faith in love takes a strong foundation to build upon. Sometimes you must dig deep before finding the foundation you need to build on. Yes, we can take shortcuts; and if we do take said shortcuts, we can expect the same results as the house not built on a firm foundation. If our love is built on shallow hearts or with shallow hearts, it will surely fall apart. The effect of such love is leaving us or others in ruins. The cause of the calamity is we settled for less love than we desire or deserve and accept subpar love. Why? Maybe we believe it is all we're going to get. Possibly it is because we deceive ourselves that we are undeserving of greater love. It could also be that we have never experienced a greater love that is agape/*Unlossable Love* from God or anyone else.

This thinking causes the individual to have a limited grasp of what they can receive from God or others. Can you imagine how much more healing could take place if they knew the healing touch of such love? Think about the foundation they can build upon for their present and future when they first build on God's love and the love of someone who not only understands such love but also lives it out!

Beatrice and Kenneth have been able to expose foster children to such love and found out many were able to heal emotionally, mentally, and even spiritually because they assisted their children to dig deep within themselves, find a solid foundation within themselves, and build trust and love on that foundation. This gives great hope for these foster children's current and future to grow where they are planted.

These are just a few examples of the cause and effects of *Unlossable Love*. There will be some who will fight this love because they fear exposing themselves to another possible failure. Their past traumas cause a realistic fear that failure with love will continue. If we live out *Unlossable Love* for these dear souls for as long as we have the opportunity; we just might enable them to experience this love for the very first time.

OVERCOMING ATTITUDES AGAINST UNLOSSABLE LOVE

Believe it or not, people sometimes fear love. As shared in the "How Does Unlossable Love Compare to Agape (Unconditional) Love?" chapter, we shouldn't fear love. Yet, because of the traumas and bad experiences of lost love, along with how some never experienced true love from someone, a person can develop a strong attitude *against the* love of any sort. Misconceptions of what love is and is not can impair one's ability to love. The effects of substances (drugs and alcohol) can alter one's perceptions of love.

The removal of emotions can definitely impair the ability to love. Believe it or not, as you enter the military, you are trained to remove the emotional element as you engage in battle because emotions can get you and others killed. Many times, this mindset is so ingrained in a person that military personnel have a very difficult time relearning how to express emotions. (This doesn't mean they have no emotions; it simply means they have a difficult time sharing their feelings with others. This is evidenced by their strong refusal to discuss feelings with others after coming back from deployments, also evidenced by the military personnel's desire to protect their family members from knowing the deep traumas they faced during deployments.) Broken trusts also contribute to the attitude of being self-imprisoned within one's mind and soul.

How can anyone overcome such traumas and difficulties and accept *Unlossable Love*? This is where the *real* work begins. It begins with the desire to heal. Too many of us want to say there's nothing wrong with us and that we're fine. We want to *appear* strong, confident, and in control. The reality is that we often suffer in silence and solitude. The appearance we project is an illusion for us to hide the wounds we suffer. I picture this like the action films where the hero is morally wounded and hides it from their love interests or their best friends and goes on as if it's just a flesh wound; that is until they die alone. They might be thinking that they are sparing their loved one's suffering when, in reality, they are robbing them of the chance to say their goodbyes and have closures. The person dying might rationalize they don't want their loved one to suffer from watching them, but the truth is they don't want them to see them in a weakened state.

Vulnerability is also a force to reckon with when addressing attitudes to overcome. Some believe that vulnerability is a weakness, and in a way they're right. Exposure, as in a battlefield experience, causes one to be apart from shielding which could protect them from harm during battle. This type of vulnerability is the most frightening to the one exposed because, at any point in time, they can be overtaken, become captive, or worse yet, casualties of the war raged upon them. Therefore, it's an attitude we must refocus on.

This same exposure can be a lifesaver for us when the right conditions are present. For this example, let's look at a surgeon doing an operation: to perform the surgery, they must expose the area in need of repair to gain access to that area. Once this takes place, the surgeon can then proceed with the healing operation on the patient. Without this vulnerability and exposure to the area in need, the patient doesn't stand a chance to receive the lifesaving care they need. The surgeon may have to cut deep, pain will be involved as part of the healing. Things that you never expected to be revealed will come to light. Pride is kicked aside, and modesty might also become submissive. These procedures are needed to bring about the healing and to remove the problem area(s) which prevent the healing. *Unlossable Love* needs the same attention and vulnerability to go deep into the person's soul and heart. God's agape/*Unlossable Love* is both the surgeon's hand and scalpel; working in harmony to carefully make the patient feel as little pain as possible. Knowing how the patient is sometimes ashamed of their exposure, God covers their shame and helps the patient to have dignity by covering them with His compassion. Here is where God repairs the brokenness, removes the cancerous elements of shame, worthlessness, and guilt, and transplants His love, forgiveness, and a healthy sense of value or self-worth, and then seals it with grace. God doesn't stop there . . .

God sends the Holy Spirit to be our ongoing therapist: causing us to follow instructions that will be healing faster and stronger than if we rely on our own skills and procedures. He will cause us to get proper rest, perform exercises that make us stronger in every manner, and be restored to our former selves (and in many ways, better than who we were!). God never leaves our sides for any reason. (Unlossable!) Yes, scars will remain. These serve two purposes: to remind us of great pains and to remind us of even greater healing!

Trust is also an effective tool for overcoming attitudes against *Unlossable Love*. Because trust has been broken, the individual has a very hard time building trust in others; God included. If a person has a broken trust (which happens to everyone), depending upon the circumstances involved, how deep the trust was broken and if the person(s) involved with breaking that trust is truly repentant of their actions, healing can either take place quickly if they attend to it quickly or it could take a great deal of healing if the person isn't sorry or care about their impact on that individual.

In the case of Beatrice and Kenneth fostering, their foster children coming into their home are coming with, in many cases, a great deal of brokenness and trust issues. These children have had promises broken by family, friends, and the foster care system; just to begin with. Add on to these possible traumas, the verbal/mental/physical/sexual abuses they witnessed or were involved with, the labels placed on them by society and peers as *"having something wrong with them"* instead of what happened to them (even those labels are equally painful and destructive); it's no wonder these children struggle as they do.

According to the CDC, it is estimated that one in seven children experience child abuse and neglect, while one in ten elders experience elder abuse and neglect. These statistics are *according to reported cases*. Many more for both categories remain unreported for unknown reasons. They are thrust into foster family homes and are "expected" to be cared for as the foster family's own. This is easy to say, but as stated earlier, building trust and rapport with some of these children is like trying to give a cat a bath; they're just not having it! Yet, when *Unlossable Love* is added to the equation, it makes it on level ground to begin to build a foundation that the children can become open to trust building.

Availability should be considered at this point. Be it a foster child, an adult, or whoever, both you and the individual need to make yourselves available to one another, and both commit to working together. Just sitting in the same room and not engaging in meaningful interaction doesn't cut it. Both need to be available to one another whenever needed. When the individual sees that you're different from the others who have let them down, their wall tumbles and you gain access to their souls. *This is a sacred trust and should be treated as such!* They will commit only as much as you are willing to commit. More than likely, it will be **you** who must prove yourself first before they will share even a small part of themselves. And depending on how much time you have together, how severe the trauma might be, and the number of years this has been going on all factor into how long it will take to discover a breakthrough with the individual(s).

Accountability can also be an effective tool for restoration. You might ask yourself, "How can accountability be an effective tool for restoration; especially when it comes to *Unlossable Love*?"

When we love someone, there is accountability for our love toward someone: if they should live up to our expectations, we continue to pour out our love toward them. On the contrary, if they should not live up to our expectations, people will rescind their love in many cases.

You may want to contradict me in this statement, however, when you look at a boyfriend or girlfriend relationship or in a marriage, you'll understand that statement recently made. We often look for individuals who can meet up to and/or exceed our expectations as we search for those whom we can invest our love into. We hold them accountable and if they cannot rise above their circumstances, we cut them out of our lives. Therefore, divorces take place, breakups continue to occur, and why relationships fall apart.

When it comes to accountability, it should not be focused on *the other person but on us.* If we are truly living out God's agape/*Unlossable Love* and if we are trying to make this our own, then it is we who are held accountable to produce and maintain that love in the individual's life. Because of the way God loves us, we understand that this is a gift from God and that it is something that can't be earned, purchased, manipulated, or coerced into being. This love exists because God deemed it so and God maintains that love for us despite ourselves and our desire to accept His love for us.

As we love in this manner, it is up to us to maintain this love for others with no preconditions or expectations. God does not force His will on us, the same can be said about His love; it simply exists and remain steadfast. If we choose to reject it, we simply don't accept it. God continues to love us despite ourselves, and He holds Himself accountable to make sure that love is completely available for us at any given time and at all times.

Acceptance—in overcoming our acceptance of *Unlossable Love*, we must make ourselves available and vulnerable enough to accept it. This is one of the hardest things for an individual to do because many of us feel that we are unredeemable and that negates us from ever "deserving" any form of love or acceptance from God or others.

This is a very sad state to be in when we believe ourselves to be unredeemable and unlovable because it blinds us to the reality that God wants to bring us into a relationship with Him and in relationships with one another. If we feel ourselves to be an outcast, we make ourselves the outcast. If we deem ourselves unlovable, then we make ourselves unlovable because we do not want to be exposed to the rejection that we presume to have from God and others. And even if we are freely receiving the agape/*Unlossable Love* from God and others, we still sometimes view ourselves as unworthy of it because of our low self-esteem and worth.

Think of the individual who has contemplated suicide: What triggers them to contemplate and attempt or succeed in their suicidal ideology? They are convinced that they are truly unlovable, unsalvageable, and unredeemable. Because of the rejection (or the perception of) acceptance and love from others (God included), the individual convinces himself or herself that their life is not worth living and that they would not be missed if they were no longer alive.

Too many times, these pre-assumptions are severely wrong and there are many who are affected by the attempt and/or completion of suicide. The individual has convinced themselves (maybe because of listening to other individuals that they have looked up to and yet have let down) that their life does not matter. The one thing about God's agape/*Unlossable Love* is that God has never let them down, nor will He ever. The individual's relationships with others here on earth, if they had only taken the time to assess their relationships with others, they would see that they are loved by more people than they thought and that their focus on their lost love was only fixated on one or a few select individuals.

Another form of acceptance that we as individuals need to focus on is our acceptance of ourselves. Throughout the years of my calling in pastoral and mental health care, I teach about this thing called self-care. Self-care is the ability to focus on and care for one's own personal needs: not just the material needs, but also the mental/emotional/physical/spiritual needs that each of us has.

This should not be misinterpreted as putting your own needs before those of others; it does mean that we are choosing to take care of ourselves in various aspects to be able to take care of others from our overflow. When a person rides in a plane, the flight attendants in their little speech before takeoff instruct us that in the case of an emergency, we are supposed to put an oxygen mask on ourselves before trying to attempt to help others. The reason for this is that if we do not take care of ourselves, we cannot help anybody else because the surrounding elements can and will overtake us and possibly destroy us.

Likewise, with self-care, we need to care for our needs and have a healthy acceptance of our own self-worth to God and to others and to ourselves to help others to live similar lives. The acceptance of our own self-worth is crucial: if we have problems accepting love, it is often an indication of low self-esteem or self-worth. The loving of ourselves opens the door for God's love to move us towards Himself where He can teach us how to appropriately love and accept love from others. It starts with us and moves outwardly. God changes the internal, which impacts the external focus to love more purely and totally.

It also goes unsaid that as we learn to be able to have acceptance for ourselves, we can educate those who struggle with this to learn ways of being able to accept love from themselves, from God, and from others. Therefore, this is the most crucial point of overcoming barriers that stand between us and *Unlossable Love*. How can we educate when we have not learned this? It is because we have learned this that we are able to show an example to those to whom we are trying to present this love, of how effective it is and transforms a life like our own.

As we live out the example of accepting love, we allow them to see the short-term and long-term effects that this love can have on each of us. People will not believe in something that we cannot believe in it ourselves; we must be convinced that this is important to us to show them how important it should be to them. This is not a form of self-righteousness or false pride, yet it is of caring enough for us that we seek the blessings of God's love and accept them with open arms.

LOVING THE UNLOVABLE

As I continue writing this book, I hear the song *There Was Jesus* by Zach Williams and Dolly Parton (piano version). Once again, I am moved to tears by the message the song delivers to my heart. In the midst of the lyrics, Zach Williams shares that in his deepest and darkest moments, there was Jesus. Throughout all his poor decisions and choices, his self-doubt and self-worthlessness, there was Jesus. He couldn't understand why He remained (Jesus) but was very thankful that He did remain.

Here was a man thinking himself unlovable and unredeemable; but the agape/*Unlossable Love* pursued him until he captured his heart, and he was restored and renewed through the love of God. I find myself within those lyrics in a time in the distant past and yet in the very presence of who I am. And even though my life has been transformed by God's love and forgiveness, Satan continues to try to confuse us and shame us out of God's love. Songs such as this remind us that once we are loved by God, he never gives up on us.

This brings me to my next point: who have we deemed unlovable in our own eyes? I can give some society-focused individuals (which I have in earlier chapters), but just the chapter title itself challenges us to probe our hearts and minds to see if there are any such ways within ourselves. Chances are, there is at least one individual or group of individuals that we can place in this category. It will be easy for us to be able to justify our thoughts about these individuals and the reasons why we think of them as unlovable. We have discussed these in the past, so we do not have to revisit the various reasons. We do have to address, though, how we respond to those that we deem "unlovable."

I invite you once again to look deep within yourself for the beginning of this response. In some form or another, there have been points in our lives when we view ourselves as unlovable. We might even think this of ourselves right now. Yet, there had been somebody in our lives either past or present who was able to share with us their love. Whether it is God or others, we were shown this love that has transformed our lives.

Personally speaking, the impact of God's love and the love of others that was shown to me in the midst of the deepest and darkest moments in my life rescued me from suicide, from my anger and rage, and assisted me to become who I am today because He was able to save (God). God brought into my life loving parents/family members, various friends, and a church body (members of the church that I attended in my youth/adulthood) that accepted me, mentor me, love me unconditionally, and help me to mature in my emotional and spiritual walk. God knew at the right time and in the right circumstances to place the right individuals to transform what I once thought was a worthless life into a precious life that is identified in Him. When I wouldn't/couldn't love myself, God provided that love in Himself and through Himself, as well as in the lives of others.

In the New Testament of the Scriptures, the apostle Paul often refers to himself as "the chief of sinners"; a self-induced statement to which he thinks himself to be the most deplorable sinner that ever walked the face of the earth. This is a term that I use for myself in many of my sermons because like Paul;

> *What then shall we say? That the law is sin? By no means! Yet if it had not been for the law, I would not have known sin. For I would not have known what it is to covet if the law had not said, "You shall not covet." But sin, seizing an opportunity through*

the commandment, produced in me all kinds of covetousness. For apart from the law, sin lies dead. I was once alive apart from the law, but when the commandment came, sin came alive and I died. The very commandment that promised life proved to be death to me. For sin, seizing an opportunity through the commandment, deceived me and through it killed me. So the law is holy, and the commandment is holy and righteous and good.

Did that which is good, then, bring death to me? By no means! It was sin, producing death in me through what is good, in order that sin might be shown to be sin, and through the commandment might become sinful beyond measure. For we know that the law is spiritual, but I am of the flesh, sold under sin. For I do not understand my own actions. For I do not do what I want, but I do the very thing I hate. Now if I do what I do not want, I agree with the law, that it is good. So now it is no longer I who do it, but sin that dwells within me. For I know that nothing good dwells in me, that is, in my flesh. For I have the desire to do what is right, but not the ability to carry it out. For I do not do the good I want, but the evil I do not want is what I keep on doing. Now if I do what I do not want, it is no longer I who do it, but sin that dwells within me. (Romans 7:7–20)

Paul is not only sharing with Romans that the law that man breaks every day (the disobedience of God's law to man) convicts us of sin, Paul is also sharing that because he is a man ("in my flesh"), the things that he wants to do for God to express his *Unlossable Love* towards God always falls short because he sees himself repetitively doing the very thing that he tries not to do.

How many of us today, and I'm especially focusing on those of us who are followers of Christ, can identify with Paul in this example? This is why I view myself like Paul to be "the chief of sinners" because I continually fail in serving God the way that I truly desire to serve Him.

Paul blames it on the sin that dwells within us; that is, sinful nature. God understands this because God fully understands us.

God knows that ever since the first sin that was created in the Garden of Eden, man's nature was corrupted. It is for this reason that the plan since before the beginning of creation, was to have Jesus present to mankind God's agape/*Unlossable Love* for the redemption and the restoration of mankind unto Himself. So, even though I view myself as this "chief of sinners", and I understand God's need and desire to love the unlovable (myself), I therefore must be able to extend that which I have learned from my own redemption to others. This is the second hardest thing to be able to do in *Unlossable Love*.

I say it is the second hardest thing to do because as we discussed earlier in the book, loving and forgiving ourselves is the first hardest act that we can do. As explained earlier, we sometimes find it much easier to forgive others and to love them and maintain a loathing for ourselves because of our awareness of who we are and what we have done in our past/present.

Just like in the movie *Spirited*, Will Ferrell's character searches to find the redemption that he had longed for. So, in the movie, his character for such an individual that was just like him and to "redeem him" to prove to himself that even someone like himself can be redeemed. Equate that redemption with love (or you can include it as part of the redemption); can we truly love someone with *Unlossable Love* when we struggle with the acceptance of it? Throughout the movie, Will's character believes himself to be unredeemable. Will is looking for an example that if it's possible for somebody else who is like him to be redeemed in the end, he too has the possibility of being redeemed in the end. Will learned throughout his time with Ryan Reynolds' character (the character that was very much like Will Ferrell's character), to build a relationship and even a "brotherhood" with Ryan's character, who in the end became redeemable.

The one thing I did not like about this particular movie is the fact that it is not our works that redeem us, but it is God who redeems us. How many of us know someone, maybe even ourselves, who believes they are unredeemable? Or how many of us are attempting to redeem ourselves by our actions? Redemption is certainly out of our capability because if they were possible, God would never have sent his son Jesus to bring the unredeemable the redemption so greatly needed to restore our intimacy with God. Man has proven to be fallible before the Infallible God. Thus, only an Infallible God can redeem the unredeemable. It is very possible, as stated earlier in the book, for God to teach us and empower us to be able to love those who are unlovable.

Throughout the Scriptures, God shows us how He is taking individuals that man has paid no attention to and has forsaken to become some of the greatest biblical examples of how God transforms lives, restores lives, and shows His agape/*Unlossable Love* towards all of mankind. Both Moses and David were murderers (David was also an adulterer), Zacchaeus was the tax collector, and both the woman at the well and the woman caught in adultery in the book of John had a very tainted past. So did Mary Magdalene, Solomon (David's son), and others at things that make people not like them very much and would even shun them. In each of these cases, God/Jesus was able to redeem their lives and transform them into living examples of God's grace and mercy in His *Unlossable Love* for us.

God investigated each of their lives and saw their potential. Knowing completely of their past and their past sins, God chose not to identify them by that past and to see the finished product of His creation in each of their circumstances. Today we can see how this approach is evidence-based and transformative in each life that it is applied. Jesus was able to transform many lives with this approach: identifying what sin is, meeting the need that the individual has, and then encouraging them to become far greater than what they are. Think about it for a moment: what if

Jesus' approach was different? How might this transform the outcomes for everyone?

Being the type of person who likes to put himself in a position to look through the eyes of different individuals, this is how I perceive it to have gone down:

- **If Jesus didn't identify the sin**—The individual might not have known that what they were doing was wrong and had caused the division between themselves and others. Today, we live in a society that does not like to hold people accountable for their actions or we have individuals who do not recognize the wrongdoing because it is socially acceptable. When this occurs, people will often keep to themselves their thoughts and feelings and allow anger and rage to compromise their ability to deal with the situation in a progressive and restoring way. That anger and bitterness place our ability to love in solitary confinement which sometimes becomes a life sentence. By Jesus identifying the sin, the situation can be dealt with once and for all, and people can be forgiven and move on toward the future which God has in store for them. If we were able to address the things that would normally separate us emotionally and spiritually, would have a more fertile ground on which we can plant the seeds of love versus trying to plant seeds within concrete.
- **Meeting the need**—God knows that man's mind is easily distracted. In order to have man's full attention, we must remove distractions. If a person comes up to me and says that they are hungry and at the same time also wants to hear the salvation story of Jesus Christ, I am not going to tell them salvation's plan before giving them something to eat. By doing so, they are distracted from hearing the message because of their hunger and then thinking about when they will get the food that they need. There are many recorded instances where people came to Jesus with

various needs. Jesus would meet those needs first and then engage with them about their relationship with God. Jesus removed the distractions to get the message across. Likewise, we should try to meet the immediate needs of the individual(s) and to relieve the distractions as much as possibly so that the individual can have more of a focus on the message of love and restoration that we are trying to share with them.

- **Encouraging them to be greater than they are (see in their potential and help them to live up to it)**—In every circumstance, Jesus never left them as He found them. After every miracle, healing, restoration, and even with those who walked away from Jesus' saving grace and restoration, Jesus would encourage them to continue in the development of their relationship with God and with one another. Those who walked away from Jesus's offer were also transformed because once we are educated about something, we cannot deny knowledge of that which is taught to us. Those individuals knew that God continually loves them with his agape/*Unlossable Love* and how it would fill the void within them; yet they chose to believe in what the world had to offer more so than what God offers to us every moment of our lives. For those who chose to live up to their potential, we can see how radically changed they have been for the better. Many of these became biblical heroes and heroines and were able to change lives themselves. The woman at the well in the book of John was able to go back to her community and because of her testimony, the entire village was able to meet and know Jesus and find salvation. In this simple act of just being able to share with them the love of God through Jesus, she was restored socially and spiritually because after having her needs met, she was able to meet the needs of others and was able to live out that example that drew others to God.

If we are truly trying to love the unlovable, we must be willing to look beyond our hurt and our pain. Sometimes, the pain is so fresh, so deep, so intense and so paralyzing that we cannot see past it. Try as we may, the pain draws us back to the focus of how deep the hurt is.

In 2008, I struck a tree in my vehicle going 55 mph. That accident caused me to have all of my ribs broken with the exception of one, a broken neck, and a broken femur, my nose was broken, my hand went through the windshield, and having multiple lacerations and bruises throughout my body. The pain from these was intense; however, the far greater pain came when they extracted me from the vehicle. Never in my life that I ever felt such physical pain and that pain caused me to yell out louder with an intensity I never knew I had within me than that moment.

Did I know that God was with me? Absolutely! Yet, at that time, I could not see past the pain. I literally had dozens of people who were working with me to not only keep me alive but to also alleviate the pain that I was in. I did not see these individuals because the pain of being extracted from the vehicle was so great. I don't remember too much after the bloodcurdling scream that I let out when being extracted from the vehicle; apart from being loaded into the helicopter which transported me to the hospital.

I share this story to give you a physical example of how pain can forbid us to see what lies ahead as far as healing and restoration because that pain is so great. Spiritually, emotionally, and mentally, those pains can have an equal effect on us. And if we have been hurt by the individual that we are trying to love, it can be extremely difficult to move past the pain. I never feared because I knew that my life was held in God's hands. I knew that whether I lived or died, I was going to be just fine because of love from God and others. Once I began my road to recovery, it didn't matter to me what my physical body shape would be: if I was ever able to walk again or be confined to a wheelchair for the rest of my life didn't faze me because I knew my value in the Lord and within those that I love and love me. Nothing of my past mattered at that moment to those who know me. My present, not my future, was first and foremost in their hearts and minds.

We shouldn't need a life-or-death experience to take place to be able to know and understand what somebody means to us or how important they are in our lives. Too often this is our reality in our present life.

Being a pastor for long as I have, and officiating over literally hundreds of funerals, I have heard over the years so many people that they were able to tell their loved ones just how much they meant to them or to be able to forgive things that they now consider to be trivial. In some cases, the last thing that the surviving family members said to the individual out of anger was "I wish you were dead!" And when that reality took place, they were unable to take those words back to be able to restore that love for that individual who had passed. This is the guilt that remains with them to this very day. Yes, they sought forgiveness from God and others, yet they still suffer. The momentary withholding of their love from the individual, in their hearts and minds, remains unforgivable.

As I counsel some of these individuals, they beg and plead to be able to take back their words and to somehow, some way be able to find a way to tell the individual who had passed of their ongoing love for them. It should never take a death or a major trauma to jar our hearts and minds to the love that we have for someone.

By nature, I believe that everyone wants to love and to be loved. We were created this way by God and when we have an absence of love, there is a void that feels as big as an eternity. If we look at God and believe in Him and what His Word says, there is nothing that can be unredeemable or unforgiving. Everything, according to God, can and will be forgiven by Him and all we must do is simply ask. And just as God knows that we will continue in our sin from time to time, His agape/*Unlossable Love* continues to fulfill His nature and forgiveness as an ongoing constant for those of us who have accepted this love. Because I believe that everyone wants to love and be loved, it is imperative that we learn that love never ends (as described in 1 Corinthians 13). When we choose to stop loving someone, I personally believe, it is because of one simple thing: we choose to love the individual with an earthly love rather than a godly love.

I will admit that there are those individuals whom I once considered to be unlovable, and I tried everything within my power to justify my hatred toward them. As you can guess, that did not work out well for me and I was the one who was doing more wrong than they were because of my anger, hatred, and bitterness that caused me to not want to give them God's love let alone my love. I was foolish to think that I was any better than they were because I know my thoughts and feelings were equally as evil and detestable in the eyes of God; thus, leaving me no room to talk about love and forgiveness. Because of God and the Holy Spirit, I've come a long way apart from that and I now know the importance of forgiveness and the love that God has for us. Every time that Satan tries to remind me of these things from my past, I share with him who I am today and because of God how I am no longer that person from my past.

Can you identify with anything thus far? Do you know where I'm coming from? As I stated before, like Paul, I am the chief of sinners. And like Paul, God's grace is sufficient. Even for me. I can't praise him enough for that grace and mercy in the way that God loves me. And like the woman at the well, I share because I have experienced the Living Water of His love. Once the outcast, now I am redeemed. There are times when I still feel that I am more of a sinner and feel that I do not deserve the grace. God reminds me through Himself and others that my worth is not determined by what I think but by whom He says I am: God's child.

Beatrice and Kenneth, along with millions of other foster parents are sometimes seen as "unlovable" by the children they foster for a different reason: *fear*. The children they foster have several reasons for fearing love and, understandably so, refrain from loving others because those who were supposed to love them had let them down and broken trusts and boundaries that they (the offenders) should never have crossed. It is natural that these children would fear risking love with someone else. Along with this, these same children long for love and when they receive it from the foster parents, they are fearful not only for the possible loss of their love; but also, because they *fear being disloyal to their biological parent(s)*. It sounds confusing to those of us who are on the outside looking in, yet there is a bond that transcends all understanding.

Foster children can experience great trauma at the hands of their biological parents which has caused Child Protective Services to step in and remove them from their parents. There are *many* factors that can cause said children to still desire connection with their biological parent; which range from being groomed by the parents, to have a mature understanding that outside influences (abusive relationships, substance abuse, for example) have caused the negative changes within the family, to their own behaviors, to mental illness and much more. *If they choose to love their foster family, these children feel as if they have betrayed their parents (whom they still deeply love), and this "guilt" is too strong to ignore and extremely difficult to deal with alongside the other circumstances they face daily.* So, the children will consider the foster family unlovable (off limits) and might act out negatively for the foster family to have a reason for not loving them. The children have justified their belief in this; even though they deeply desire the love they are receiving from the foster family.

Adults also use this method to prevent being victimized by others. They might consider those of us "unlovable" because their fear is so intense of being hurt again. We sometimes believe this of ourselves: if we don't love ourselves and make ourselves unlovable, we "control" the depth of pain allowed. What we fail to see is that as we do this, our self-isolation becomes cancerous and kills us gradually. Before we know it, there's no hope for us unless we go to the Great Physician Jesus Christ, who can and does cure us as we seek his healing touch on our hearts.

As stated earlier, love is a choice: we choose to love or reject love (or shall I clarify this by saying the impact on our lives). Real *Unlossable Love* is never limited and those who love this way will testify that *nothing* we do can change our love or God's love for us. We can and do limit its effectiveness by not receiving it and utilizing it to transform our hearts. We can't force someone to accept our love, but we can show them that they don't have to remain unlovable. We can assist them to overcome their fears by sharing with them they can love others *and* love their biological family at the same time; that they themselves have that deep love within themselves. Finally, they have the power to create the love they have so longed for and to empower them to make their world a greater place because *their love* can become the *Unlossable Love* they long for.

NOT FAKING IT TILL YOU MAKE IT; ACTUALLY LOVING THE PERSON(S)

Many of us have heard (and possibly used) the term, "Fake it till you make it." I don't know about you, but this is sometimes a very disturbing statement to make. Ponder upon this statement for a moment and consider each term used in it: Fake it till you make it. To me, it's an oxymoron; like jumbo shrimp, it doesn't make sense.

Return to the days of your youth for a moment—then maybe you and a sibling or friend get into a fight. The parents or grown-ups present force you to say you're both sorry to one another. One or both of you *really aren't sorry*; in fact, you might have wished you could have continued the fight. However, the adults' presence forces us to make up and play nice.

So, we reluctantly say we're sorry and stay away from one another. Maybe we really made up later in the days or weeks to come and maybe we still haven't made up and the battle rages on within us. But if you faked it till you made it, did others see the fakeness in our apologies? Could others tell that we didn't really mean it and wanted the battle to continue until we destroyed our opponents? Chances are, they did see it.

Let's take a deeper look into this situation: what did you feel during that time? A great number of factors can influence your thoughts and feelings. What these factors are can differ from one to another. Social norms, cultural influences, family dynamics, traumatic experiences (not necessarily directed towards the individual, but also include events such as 9/11, experiencing an act of violence or accident, etc.), and connections to a faith system all play a part in how one responds to an event and their resilience to the situation one is involved with. These can either make one more prone to deal with their circumstances or impair their abilities to respond. When I ask, "What did you feel at the time?" a person can respond to the situation one time just fine and differently to a similar incident. Or, a person, if this occurs repeatedly to them, can lose their ability to adjust or address the circumstance properly because they are weakening due to the ongoing actions taking place. Like a battery, if we continually use its resources, the battery sooner or later dies. So it is with our emotions, feelings, and desire to persevere.

Now, addressing the "fake it" aspect of loving someone. *Unlossable Love* doesn't know how to fake it; it's all in or not at all (at least for mankind). God's agape/*Unlossable Love* is ALWAYS all in! Think for a moment: Does God ever "fake it to make it"? If this was possible for God, how would it make you feel that God was faking His love for you, and you knew about it?

As I was working in the mental health field, those whom I served could tell right off the bat if you invested in their lives by the way you reacted and interacted (or lack thereof) with them. I recall a certain girl who was 14 years old that I began to work with. She was *so* broken; she caused all sorts of disruptions and chaos during her therapy sessions that some of her therapists were in tears during or after sessions with her.

I was assigned to her case for special classes for her. And, as you can guess, she fought me every step of the way. The more I worked with her, the more she would try to drive me away from her. I told her that she could trust in me and that I truly cared for her. Her response to me was, *"You only care for me because you're paid to care for me!"*

I looked at her and responded, "Honey, you can tell that I care for you because with what you're doing, they can't pay me enough to go through what I do with you!" At first, she took it like a badge of honor; thinking that she was wearing me down. She underestimated one thing: God was involved and had different plans for her!

Time went on and she began to realize I was steadfast in my relationship with her. This scared her because she couldn't manipulate me like she had the others, she couldn't bully me away from her like she did the therapists, and she was confused why I didn't back off like the others. I would always share with her that if she ever wanted to talk, I would make myself available for her. She couldn't believe me at first. She *didn't want to believe* me (as we discussed in the last session) because she had such traumatic experiences happen to her that she was afraid to allow anyone to get close to her again.

One night, she was involved in an incident which had changed everything between us. She was involved in this situation in which, in her words, she was having a total meltdown and she was going off the deep end. Through the grace of God (and He alone gets the glory for this), she remembered that I promised her that she could call me at any time, and I would respond. She had told her mother and stepfather that she wanted to talk with me amid her raging outburst. Her stepfather said to her, "He doesn't want to talk with you; he's only paid to talk with you. It's after hours and he probably won't answer the phone."

She insisted on talking to me, so the stepfather wanted to prove himself right and called me. He stated that she wanted to talk with me and that she was "out of control."

I instructed him to hand her the phone. She went on to share with me the incident that had taken place and we talked for about two hours. At the end of the conversation, she was a great deal calmer and she had promised me that she would talk with me the next day, and she did.

In the weeks to come, I noticed a dramatic change in her interactions with me: She was more attentive to the lessons, she engaged more

Not Faking It till You Make It; Actually Loving the Person(s)

in the sessions, she was getting deeper in conversations, and she believed in what I had to share.

She shared with me that day on which I spoke with her during her crisis that it was a turning point for her. She went on to explain that she knew on that night that my caring for her was real, and she realized I was in it for her and not because I was being paid. She continued to say if I hadn't connected with her that evening that she had plans for taking her own life because she couldn't live like that anymore. She went from being my number one disrupter to becoming my greatest reason for being at the facility.

I truly believe that God had empowered me to see her true brokenness and used me as part of her healing and restoration. She had seen that I didn't fake it but that I truly loved her as one of my own children and loved her with an *Unlossable Love* which God had provided for her. To this day, we are still in contact with one another. She credits me for changing her life around, but I must give it to God alone because he placed me to be working with her and empowered me to remain steadfast in my commitment to her.

This new woman recently texted me and, in our conversation, she again stated that her progress in life is because of me. I stated that she had done all the work on her own. She responded that if someone else was leading the group at the time, she never would have done the work. She claims I was able to assist her in finding a reason for the change, for living, and to see life in a different and better light. I told her that it was God that brought us together and she was thankful that she can see this now. She now has a sweet little girl of her own and she is thankful for all she has.

Again, I write this not in boasting of myself, but to boast for the Lord God who made all this happen. Can you imagine how the outcome would have been different if she thought I was just faking it? When we say we're going to do something, people will hold us to our words.

And if we were "faking it till we make it", our façade would have been exposed and great calamity would have taken place. Instead, God was able to restore her life to the way she now desires it to be for herself and her daughter. It takes actual love to make actual differences in the lives of others! There are no shortcuts or ways around this. Jesus took this seriously enough to take it all the way to the cross. We shouldn't commit to anything less.

A person might believe they can fool people with their "love," but it is always a matter of time before that is exposed for what it truly is or isn't. Those who are prone to produce domestic violence toward others know exactly what they're doing as they search for their next victim. They know how to charm and convince their targets into believing that they have found the perfect significant other: they will "love" them, care for them and help their targets to gain a false sense of daydream life with them before turning it into a nightmare. They make the changes in small ways and, if you're not watching out for it, become more selfish with you being with others. They begin to isolate you and demand more of your time. They continue by tearing apart relationships that you have and making you focus on the fact that your relationship with them is the most important relationship to focus on. They become more controlling and if you don't meet their expectations, they "put you in your place."

By this time, all is exposed and what you thought was love at first is now a controlling factor. This doesn't happen to everyone; but if it happens to just one person, that's one too many. Their "fake it till you make it" is more of a trap; like the Venus flytrap; it lures its prey with sweet nectar, and it leads to the death of its prey.

Even if your intent is honorable and you don't plan on harming the individual(s), faking love can and will have devastation that you never anticipated. If you're discovered to be faking your love, it could make the individual you are doing this with withdraw emotionally, doubt their self-worth or value, feel like you were playing them for a fool, and

Not Faking It till You Make It; Actually Loving the Person(s)

break the trust which they placed in the relationship. The only way to avoid this is to *make your love genuine and real.*

Love is a choice. Love also is demanding; yet not in the way one might believe. When I say love is demanding, real love demands to grow and continually reach out. Like strawberry plants, love is invasive and wants to take over its host. One can't love only part way. If God only loved us part way, Jesus never would have done what He did for our salvation. Numerous miracles would never have taken place. Evil would have a stronger hold on the world than it does today. God IS love and His Nature causes Him to never give up on His love towards us. God purposely loves us because of who He is.

I don't know about you, but I *can't* fake love. I'm terrible at faking this! I am a good actor at times (at least in my own mind), but something this serious in nature, I take very seriously. Because of my upbringing and experiences, I couldn't ever desire to fake love because I had it done unto me, and, let me tell you, it is the most terrible experience to go through when you believe you're loved; only to be made a fool. Because of how God had restored me and my ability to love; adding the fact that these experiences had shown me the importance of not faking love with others,

I take love *very* seriously. Earlier in this book, we discussed the various ways people love. If I tell you that I love you, it is the real deal and not founded on worldly love! I don't use the word love without realizing the expectation that goes along with the use of love. When I love, I love with *Unlossable Love,* and if I love you in this way, the only way my love changes is to continually grow with the grace of God. I *choose* to love this way because this is the way God taught me how to love. He can and will do the same for you if you desire this for yourself.

This doesn't mean that you won't make mistakes from time to time. This means that you will love one another enough to work through your difficulties with this love. This love means you will never give up on loving and caring for this individual. It will take you out of your comfort zone when you least expect it and for longer than anticipated. This love means vulnerability and transparency. It might keep you up at night worrying about your loved ones. It will move you to do things that never entered your mind. It means loving individuals whom others (or yourself) might deem unlovable and/or unredeemable, but God has placed this person on your heart to be their changing agent in life. This is a great responsibility; it's also a humbling opportunity for God to use us to bring hope and restoration to those around us.

You don't have to fake it to make it when it comes to *Unlossable Love*. Love is never pretending there is absolutely no way to fake it. Real love is as obvious as the sun in the morning and the moon at night. You know that it is there, you know that it continues even when you can't see it, and you know when you are touched by it. As we learn our role in how this plays out in our own lives and the lives of others, we begin to realize that we want our love to be as real as God's love toward us.

PERSONAL, SPIRITUAL, AND MENTAL/EMOTIONAL IMPACTS OF UNLOSSABLE LOVE

Unlossable Love is transformational in the life of those who embrace it. This love affects us in every aspect of our life, and I believe that it would be a good time to investigate just how. Throughout the book, we have discussed what this love is, where its origins came from, how to develop it within ourselves, having the ability to use it on ourselves and with others, and in some ways how it can impact an individual. It's now time to go deeper into the effects that *Unlossable Love* has on someone like me.

As I shared at the beginning of the book, when Beatrice shared the name of this love and began to describe to me what it was according to her, I literally had goose bumps all over my body. That was an instantaneous response to discover how such love exists. And throughout our time together, I began to realize that this love isn't anything new, but that it was something that God has established long before he created man. The further I dove into understanding this love from God, the more it became apparent to me the necessity for me to bring this to light so that others may see what I have been experiencing.

I've had many personal experiences and have knowledge of other people's experiences as they shared with me their ongoing struggles, lack of self-worth, lack of hope, and feeling unredeemable. Because I'm very much human and have emotions like everyone else, the same doubts and fears arose in my heart on numerous occasions: what if I'm not good enough and I will always be a screw-up? God's agape/*Unlossable Love* has shown me that it has nothing to do with me being "good enough" and is not based on my works. His love towards me is founded in His love for me. At all my darkest moments, God's love was abundantly clear and His presence unmistakable. God had placed in my life the right people at the right time for the right purpose for me to become who I am today. Seeing this from hindsight enables me to write what I do today with the assurance of that which I'm sharing now. I know that if God was not there for me when I needed him most with the love that He has, I never would've been restored and renewed. My confidence is not found within me, but it is founded in the truths of who God is to me.

I have already shared several instances throughout this writing about how God has and always will continue His agape/*Unlossable Love* for me so that I may mirror and reflect this same love towards others like yourselves. It is evidence-based in me how effective this love is. Beatrice and Kenneth, through their foster care and own personal family, have shown the effectiveness of this love from those whom they care for. I shared with you in the previous chapter about the young lady whose life was changed because of *Unlossable Love* and she is now living the life that she has always longed for because of it.

We've already discussed how love is a choice: how we accept it and to whom we give it. We've had discussions on the importance of continuation and steadfastness in this love and how this real love if it is as real as we believe it to be, cannot be contained or manipulated. When we make this love personal to us, we open ourselves to be personal with others; allowing them to be drawn in by this love so that they may receive his healing touch and all the beauty that it holds. I know how personally I am blessed that Beatrice was able to share with me that which God has placed on her heart. I am humbled and blessed that that love would motivate me to write this book and to share with you all that I have learned so that you may be blessed by God. Both Beatrice and I give this glory to God and to God alone.

We gain a personal impact from *Unlossable Love* when we *make it personal: by either receiving this love or giving it.* I've always said that it isn't personal until we make it personal.

I had just returned from doing pastoral visitation with several parishioners who are homebound. In our communication, we discussed the various changes we have seen over the decades in our society, technology, theology, and other areas of change. As we talked, we compared today's generation's mindset versus our generation's thought process. What we discovered is that each generation has some things the other doesn't understand about the other because we're not taking the time to get to know one another and learn from one another. One of the older men I spoke with shares in our conversation, "My wife and I don't do as much volunteering as we use to not only because we're older, but the young folks can take over."

This then led to discussions about our "callings" (how God calls us to serve in specific ways) and how some people choose not to serve in charitable organizations. I had shared that statement about how it's not personal until it's *personal*; that unless we are directly affected, we often don't care as much. However, when we are directly affected, it becomes very personal. I used a story from that day's news that talked about strong storms and tornadoes down south, sharing that as we hear these stories, we can have a sense of sorrow or concern for those involved. The gentleman stated that he felt the same way, but it was not a heavy burden because he is far removed from the situation. He added that if it had happened here where he lives, the impact would greatly differ from the initial response of the distant storm coverage.

This opened the door to discussing how certain people are called to serve in different ways *because of the personal connection and experiences we become subject to.* I have a *strong* passion for those who are broken, abandoned, forgotten, and for youth. This is because I was once in their shoes and when God brought others into my life to make a difference, God mentored me to develop the heart of not only a pastor but after Christ's own heart.

Not everyone can understand our calling because they have never walked in our shoes. I am passionate because of my experiences. Moses, from the Old Testament, witnessed the cruel and inhumane treatment of God's people (Hebrews) and this caused him (Moses) to kill the guard who inflicted the harsh treatment. Moses, who was a Hebrew by birth, realized that something had to be done and the rest is history. (For more on this story, read the book of Exodus in the Scriptures.) It became personal.

This is a good segue for discussion of the spiritual impact of *Unlossable Love*. The discussion about how God is the Author of this love has already taken place. A great example from the Bible is as follows:

> *He entered Jericho and was passing through.* **And** *behold, there was a man named* **Zacchaeus**. *He was a chief tax collector and was rich. And he was seeking to see who Jesus was, but on account of the crowd he could not, because he was small in stature. So he ran on ahead and climbed up into a sycamore tree to see him, for he was about to pass that way. And when Jesus came to the place, he looked up and said to him, "Zacchaeus, hurry and come down, for I must stay at your house today." So he hurried and came down and received him joyfully. And when they saw it, they all grumbled, "He has gone in to be the guest of a man who is a sinner." And* **Zacchaeus** *stood and said to the Lord, "Behold, Lord, half of my goods I give to the poor. And if I have defrauded anyone of anything, I restore it fourfold." And Jesus said to him, "Today salvation has come to this house, since he also is a son of Abraham. For the Son of Man came to seek and to save the lost.*[8]

---

[8] *The Holy Bible: English Standard Version* (Lk 19:1–10). (2016). Crossway Bibles.

Personal, Spiritual, and Mental/Emotional Impacts of Unlossable Love

Zacchaeus was a man who was despised because he was a tax collector who was looked down upon (not because of his height but because tax collectors in those days would overcharge the people and keep the profits). He had heard stories about this man named Jesus and Jesus had come to his town. Because he was so short, he had to climb a tree just to catch a glimpse of the Lord. As you read the story of how Jesus showed Zacchaeus agape/*Unlossable Love*, Zacchaeus was a changed man both socially and spiritually as evidenced by his repentant heart and actions in making things right.

There is a spiritual impact from *Unlossable Love*. The Scriptures are full of examples of transformed lives once the individual has made the personal intimacy with God/Jesus/Holy Spirit. When God connects, lives are transformed, mostly for the better (I say this because there are times when God would connect with someone, and they would reject the relationship with Him.) Yet another example of this is again found in the book of Luke:

> *One of the criminals who were hanged railed at him, saying, "Are you not the Christ? Save yourself and us!" But the other rebuked him, saying, "Do you not fear God, since you are under the same sentence of condemnation?* ***And*** *we indeed justly, for we are receiving the due reward of our deeds; but this man has done nothing wrong." And he said, "Jesus, remember me when you come into your kingdom." And he said to him, "Truly, I say to you, today you will be with me in paradise." (Luke 23:39–43)*

Two criminals, one on each side of Jesus, are crucified. Both criminals had the same opportunity as the other to either receive or reject Jesus in their final moments. Jesus would have offered the same thing to each, yet only one accepted while the other rejected. One mocked and the other protected. One sought to produce emotional pain while the other sought intimacy with Jesus in his (the criminal's) last moment; even though this thief had nothing to offer in return. We see Jesus respond the only way God would respond: with agape/*Unlossable Love*. As this criminal took his last breath here on earth, his next breath was in paradise with Jesus.

I would also like to share as far as the spiritual aspect of it on how reassuring it is that God loves us so much with his agape/*Unlossable Love* that He is willing to forgive us when we have deliberately disrespected Him and continually tries to restore us back into the intimate relationship that he desires to have with each of us. Jesus tells us the story in the form of a parable (a parable is an exaggerated story to be able to share an important truth):

> *And he said, "There was a man who had two sons. And the younger of them said to his father, 'Father, give me the share of property that is coming to me.' And he divided his property between them. Not many days later, the younger son gathered all he had and took a journey into a far country, and there he squandered his property in reckless living. And when he had spent everything, a severe famine arose in that country, and he began to be in need. So he went and hired himself out to one of the citizens of that country, who sent him into his fields to feed pigs. And he was longing to be fed with the pods that the pigs ate, and no one gave him anything.*
>
> *"But when he came to himself, he said, 'How many of my father's hired servants have more than enough bread, but I perish here with hunger! I will arise and go to my father, and I will say to him, "Father, I have sinned against heaven and before you. I am no longer worthy to be called your son. Treat me as one of your hired servants."' And he arose and came to his father. But while he was still a long way off, his father saw him and felt compassion, and ran and embraced him and kissed him. And the son said to him, 'Father,*

Personal, Spiritual, and Mental/Emotional Impacts of Unlossable Love

I have sinned against heaven and before you. I am no longer worthy to be called your son.' But the father said to his servants, 'Bring quickly the best robe, and put it on him, and put a ring on his hand, and shoes on his feet. And bring the fattened calf and kill it, and let us eat and celebrate. For this my son was dead, and is alive again; he was lost, and is found.' And they began to celebrate.

"*Now his older son was in the field, and as he came and drew near to the house, he heard music and dancing. And he called one of the servants and asked what these things meant. And he said to him, 'Your brother has come, and your father has killed the fattened calf, because he has received him back safe and sound.' But he was angry and refused to go in. His father came out and entreated him, but he answered his father, 'Look, these many years I have served you, and I never disobeyed your command, yet you never gave me a young goat, that I might celebrate with my friends. But when this son of yours came, who has devoured your property with prostitutes, you killed the fattened calf for him!' And he said to him, 'Son, you are always with me, and all that is mine is yours. It was fitting to celebrate and be glad, for this your brother was dead, and is alive; he was lost, and is found.'" (Luke 15:11–16)*

In this parable, Jesus is sharing a particular story with the crowd around Him. Jesus is trying to point out the importance of everyone being able to be restored into an intimate relationship by God the Father. Like the father in the story, God will give us our heart's desires; even if He knows the great harm that it could bring. I am sure that the father in the story tried to talk some sense into his youngest son, but the son simply did not want to pay attention to what his father had to say.

This is very much like many of us today; God is trying to protect us from great catastrophes and traumas when He asks us to follow

His directions and we believe that we have everything figured out and might even think that we know more than God.

As the story unfolds, we realize that the son squandered all the blessings that his father gave him on a frivolous lifestyle. When those resources are exhausted, the son finds himself in a deplorable state and he begins to realize who his father is and what a blessing his father is. The son then tries to return home with the thought that he would only be a servant because his father would reject him for disrespect and disregard of his directions. And, just like God, the story reveals how the father was forever vigilant each day, eagerly awaiting the son's return home. When the father saw his son returning home, he ran out to meet him and immediately embraced him. Before the son could even attempt to say a word, the father called for his servants to bring forth all the different things that indicated that this young man was his son: the family robe and the family ring.

I share the story because I find great comfort spiritually knowing that when I make poor choices and mistakes, and I go prodigal for however long I may, when I come back home to God and asked to restore the relationship between us, God will greet me in the same way as this father greeted his son. And there's an important factor that would like to add to this point: others may not agree with our Heavenly Father's approach.

In the story, the prodigal son's brother stayed by his father's side and did what the father requested. When he found out all that his father had done for his wayward brother, the older brother got very upset. Understandable that he would be upset, but it doesn't give him the right to be upset. The father went on to say that everything that the older brother had done was duly noted and that he would definitely receive all of the blessings and honor that is bestowed on him by the father. At the same time, the father put the older son in his place and shared with him the importance of having his brother back home once again.

Personal, Spiritual, and Mental/Emotional Impacts of Unlossable Love

Today, we might have the same attitude or mindset as the older brother when we see such injustice taking place and think that those involved haven't had "real consequences" for their actions. We believe that they need to know the pain they've caused others. I am so thankful God is like the father in the story of Jesus; He (God) doesn't give us what we deserve, but He gives us what we need. This makes me spiritually drawn to the love of the Father. I can see God's agape/*Unlossable Love* at work in the son's restoration.

The mental and emotional aspects of *Unlossable Love* are linked together in the same way twins are connected: both are separate and joined as mirror images. Emotions affect the mental stability and health of the individual. Mental health can also affect how one perceives and responds to emotions. For the sake of discussion, let us focus first on the emotions.

> *Emotions are at the core of our being and reflect one profound aspect of the wonder of being made in the image of God (Num. 32:10; Is. 53:3; John 11:33). More than anything else they reflect our attitudes and behavior. Emotions often express outwardly our innermost beliefs. For instance, if we believe in God's sovereignty and ultimate control, we exchange fear and worry for peace and contentment.*
>
> *God makes Himself known to us not only in truth and by decree but in the way He reveals His heart. God is passionate in His pursuit of us, and that passion is expressed in a variety of **emotions**: grief at the rebellion of His children (Hos. 11:8, 9), anger at their idolatry (Jer. 2:11–13), and delight upon their return to Him (Luke 15:11–32). God's longing for an unhindered relationship with His children is found all through Scripture (Jer. 17:9, 10).*
>
> *Women, too, who **are** made in His image not only think and choose—they feel. Their personalities **are** interwoven with an intricate mix of mind, will, and **emotions**. To be able to experience pain*

or joy, sadness or anger is to feel alive. You not only do yourself damage and limit your potential in Christ when you deny or suppress your emotions, you reduce your understanding of who God is. Emotion—that is passionate, heartfelt desire—is part of the energy that bonds believers to God and to each other in a rich, meaningful way. See also Ex. 15:1–18; Ps. 66:1–20; Nahum 1:6, 7; Eph. 5:25–32; notes on Anger (Eccl. 7); Depression (1 Sam. 16); Grief (Is. 53); Healing (Ps. 13); Mental Health (John 10)[9]

I believe emotions serve mankind as a form of protection as well as to express the feelings within. Emotions not only express the feelings one might have; they also serve as warning signs that help us to avoid problems. If we are anxious about something, it might mean that God is trying to warn us not to do something. Some might call it a conscience; I call it the leading of the Holy Spirit.

When this occurs, I pay close attention! (I will admit that sometimes, like the younger son in the story, I can be just as much of a knucklehead as he was!) Emotions can protect us from placing ourselves in harmful situations, provide joy when we make good choices, help us to express fears and anxieties, and cause us to slow down and be cautious.

Is it possible to have good mental health and be emotional at the same time? Yes. Is it possible if it were the other way around? Yes. If so, then what effect does *Unlossable Love* have on these elements?

Unlossable Love is the stabilization of emotions and mental health. If we are to become out of control for whatever reason, we can turn to this love and find reasoning and comfort as we rationally search for the answers we need at that time. Our emotions sometimes cause us to overreact and believe in the worst-case scenarios for our circumstances.

---

9 Patterson, Dorothy Kelly, et. al., *The Woman's Study Bible*. (Nashville: Thomas Nelson, 1995).

Personal, Spiritual, and Mental/Emotional Impacts of Unlossable Love

Our emotions can confuse us to the point where we can develop a mental illness: depending on the severity of the situation. If we can understand we are loved regardless of our mistakes, it can bring great relief from the guilt of losing something so dear to us. Some might look at this and think it gives the person a license to continue in their behaviors and choices. However, like in the prodigal story, it moved the son to repentance and restoration.

Please note that the success of this is the *consistency* of those around the individual seeking the restoration. The father was consistent with his vigil for his son to return and he was consistent with his love for his son. (Remember how we discussed the importance of love being real and not faking it till you make it?) God's consistency is vital for our recovery. Likewise, our love towards others must also mirror God's love. This is an evidence-based practice that is time-proven and will be throughout eternity. The more consistent we are in our love, the greater the chance for the individual(s) to find the *Unlossable Love* we write about.

WHEN A PERSON TRIES TO RUN FROM UNLOSSABLE LOVE

What? Who in their right mind would *ever* want to run from the *Unlossable Love* that you've been sharing? You might be thinking this after reading the title of this chapter. Believe it or not, this is a reality for many. If *Unlossable Love* is everything we say it is (and it is!), why then would anyone run from it?

There could be many different possibilities, and we will discuss some within this chapter. It is all about the individual, the various traumas and experiences, supports or lack thereof, the genuineness of the love given to the individual, and the consistency of that love and support which will determine the overall outcome for *Unlossable Love*. I will share several reasons which I have personally experienced; along with some from which those I have assisted in the past have shared with me their reasons.

Loss—This is a broad statement for a reason because what looks like a loss to one might not be a loss for another. This doesn't discount either one's understanding. An example of this is the loss of a pet. To one person, the death of a pet, if the pet runs away, or if the pet is given to another because of something like moving into a new home where pets aren't allowed; the loss could be thought of as, "It's just an animal; it isn't that important . . . " To someone else, that pet might have become part of the family and the bond with the animal is strong. When I lost my *favorite* cat Mordecai to death, I lost a best friend and family member. I grieved (and continue after several years) and mourned his death. I have had other pets that died, and I never did shed a tear for them.

Children entering the foster care system lose plenty of multiple losses at the same time: being taken away from their biological family, their schools change, they have to leave their pets, their physical homes, their friends, their churches or faith systems, their traditions, and even their cultures and identity as they enter the foster family's home. Yes, many of these foster parents are sensitive to these needs, yet to the children; depending on their ages and experiences, they have lost *everything* (And in most cases, they have!)

So naturally, when *Unlossable Love* is introduced, the children "turn off" their feelings or rejects anyone who tries to get in a close relationship with them because who's to say that it won't happen again?

Rejection—Similar to loss; rejection is crueler and has a deeper impact on the individual. The pain inflicted by rejection has created irrational thought processes to go into overdrive and those who are rejected can (and do) make extremely poor choices, which could also lead to suicidal ideations and possibly suicide completions. For those of us who have/had young teenagers who started dating and "broke up," how did they respond and react? If your children were like mine; they thought the world had come to an end and life wouldn't go on without their significant other being their soulmate. Regardless of age, such rejections have destroyed a vast number of lives emotionally, mentally, and even spiritually.

The rejection doesn't have to be that abrupt to have the same effects on a person. In my case, as I was going through my issues with my parents (my father especially), their inability to support me in my various stages in life in the same ways they did two of my other brothers, I felt rejected because my interests differed than my two brothers and my father. I tried to earn my father's attention and affection, but he never supported me in the same manner as he did my brothers. He never went to my play at school, the numerous band performances, or even my wedding! I never thought I ever mattered to him unless he was drunk. I never heard him say to me personally that he was ever proud of me. (I am not sharing this for a "poor me" session, but to explain what it felt like as I went through what we did together at that time.)

Fortunately for me, as I became older and wiser and I addressed it with my father, I discovered many of the barriers *he had to work through* while we were going through it. It was a gradually perceived rejection that intensified throughout the years, and it had a profound impact on our relationship as father and son.

Grooming—There are people who are gifted and persuasive and who know just how to manipulate others to gain control of the individuals they target. Normally, those who are considered as being narcissistic, sociopathic, or psychopathic are considered to be the best at this form of control. They groom others to follow their (the groomer's) needs and desires. They will convince the individual(s) how deeply they love and care for you, and before you know it, they have their hooks deep in your heart and begin to control every aspect of your life.

I share this with you because if these individuals are effective in their schemes, they can manipulate the minds and hearts of others. We see evidence of this in cults where they convince the individual(s) to leave homes and relationships to serve in their cult. Once groomed, they can and do convince the individual(s) to do things that they would have never considered before. It takes a great deal of deprogramming these lost souls to see the realities they had placed themselves in. These cults promise the people instant acceptance of who they are and how they will protect them from all harm. They gain their trust and after they are conditioned, they begin to slowly introduce their wishes for the people to serve them. They begin to also isolate the people from their loved ones, sharing how they have held them back from joy and peace. If the individual(s) are weak-minded or if their past traumas are severe enough, they will do whatever is asked because of their desire to belong and to be loved. They promise *Unlossable Love* and fail to deliver it.

Lack of understanding—In this arena, understanding is a double-edged sword: both the individual and the others involved in the individual(s) life can possibly have a lack of understanding. The individual believes or perceives the impressions that they are misunderstood and that others refuse to understand or can't understand the individual. As this occurs, the individual becomes angered and frustrated at their situation, and the lack of understanding on the part of those whom they seek *Unlossable Love*. This causes those involved in the relationship to have a failure to communicate properly and the understanding they seek never occurs.

Foster children, those who have experienced trauma (personally done towards them or observed), dysfunctional families, veterans, first responders, those in the medical fields; even clergy and morticians, and a host of others have exposure to events and situations which we (the individual) believe are unique to themselves. As we begin to share our experiences, it often becomes apparent that those we share with haven't a clue what it feels like to be in such circumstances. Try as we may assist those to gain understanding, it falls on deaf hearts. Yes, they might try to go through the motions of active listening and God bless them for it. However, if we feel that no one can understand our situations and how this has distanced us from others, we simply close our mouths and keep our brokenness and anger to ourselves.

In 2004, my then 18 yr. old daughter gave birth to conjoined twins. The story made national news. Two months into the pregnancy, my daughter was encouraged to have an abortion by her physicians; stating that the twins, IF they were born, wouldn't survive more than just moments outside the womb. My daughter stated that she wouldn't get the abortion and she carried her twin daughters to birth. Rebecca and Stephanie McCray were born on January 20th and died on January 24th; four days longer than anyone expected. During these four days, my daughter and the rest of our family and friends were able to give Rebecca and Stephanie *Unlossable Love*—the girls know what it is like to be loved and touched with love and care from their families. They heard their mother's voice and felt her kisses. Their aunt and uncle also shared their love for them. And of course, Nana and Pappaw also loved on both Rebecca and Stephanie for as long as they could. Why do I share this? To prove a point.

As their grandfather (Pappaw), and a pastor, I was asked to give Rebecca and Stephanie an anointing and to Baptist them literally moments after their birth. Can you imagine what that felt like for someone like me? Throughout Rebecca's and Stephanie's life for the next four days, my daughter and our family went through a lot of emotions, hope and hopelessness, joys, and sorrows, and yet ALL were and are blessings at the same time. All of this, while dealing with the media covering the story, being a pastor and doing my pastoral duties, being a parent and grandparent walking with the family through this experience. Needless to say, at the time of Rebecca's and Stephanie's funeral, we had literally THOUSANDS of people sharing their condolences and trying to share how they knew what we were going through. REALLY? I mean, we did and do truly appreciate the love and support during our time of Rebecca's and Stephanie's passing; but to be honest with you, their birth was literally more than one in a million birth and the fact they survived outside the womb for as long as they did is more than a miracle! None of my many pastor friends could identify with us and our situation. Like I had shared earlier, when we understood that no one could identify with us, we graciously accepted their *Unlossable Love* and their beautiful gifts of support for what they were.

Just recently, 18 years later, I was watching an episode of *Yellowstone*. In this episode, there was a loss of an infant child. Kevin Costner's character was consoling the child's mother (his daughter-in-law). This is what he said to her:

When a Person Tries to Run from Unlossable Love

> *"That boy lived a perfect life, Monica. We're the only ones who knew it was brief. All he knew was you and that you loved him."*

As I watched it, it brought me back to when Rebecca and Stephanie were born, lived, and died. I wish I had these words back then and I promise I will forever use these when I work with families who have lost infants to death. These words were beautifully said and reflected to me that whoever wrote this can and did identify with our loss! Of course, I and my wife wept as we watched it in the *Yellowstone* episode. This time, the weeping was a precious gift of joy.

When we try to run from *Unlossable Love*, it always finds a way to reach us. In my circumstance with Rebecca and Stephanie, it took 18 years to connect with someone who truly understands. Those simple words brought a beautiful crescendo to an already blessing. God, with His agape/*Unlossable Love*, reaches out to all of us and tries to help us to understand that we don't have to run from Him and those whom He brings into our lives. How do we know which ones He brings into our lives versus those who try to infiltrate our life? God makes abundantly clear those whom He places in our lives to help us. We sometimes might not see this because we are fighting to run away from getting close to others or to God and our fear of getting hurt again creates this fear. God refuses to be silent, and He will do everything to make us aware of His love for us. The choice is then ours to either accept or decline His love. Even when we reject this blessing, He continues to remain faithful to us until we either accept His gift or draw our last breath here on earth.

WHEN OUR SOURCE OF UNLOSSABLE LOVE DIES— THE IMPACT

Just the other day, I was speaking to my friend Paul. We have been friends for over 40 years and our story is a lasting friendship that started back in high school. During this time, I have moved from Rhode Island (my home state and where I met Paul) to Wisconsin, back to Rhode Island, and to where I live now in Indiana. We have kept in touch all those years and EVERY TIME my family went out east to New England, we always made plans to at least have a meal together with Paul and his family. As we were talking on the phone the other day, we talked about our friendship and for whatever reason, the discussion of people dying came into the conversation. Paul told me, "If anything ever happened to you (if I would die), I would lose it big time! I don't know what I would do without you in my life…".

The reasoning for such a statement is because he has received and continues to receive *Unlossable Love* from myself and my family. When we look at this; we can identify this feeling and thought process with those we love dearly. Children feel this way with their parents (if the relationship is a healthy relationship), spouses also feel this way with one another, and so on. I wish that I could promise those I love that I will always be there to love them the way I do. Yet, someday, I will die. I might move away from the area and the current ways we engage with one another will change. I may not be able to meet the needs of others in the ways I would like to, or they desire me to meet their needs. What happens then?

This is a tough question with no textbook answer: each relationship and response differ from one person to the next, circumstances can intensify and cause a chasm between individuals and irrational thought processes can overtake rational truths, fears can distort our perception of the situation, and outside influences can manipulate the situation. In all cases mentioned, the result remains the same: the source of our *Unlossable Love* dies; metaphorically or physically. This can and does have a profound effect on those left behind. What is the proper way to address such a loss?

Over the course of 22 years of being a pastor, I have officiated literally hundreds of funerals, memorial services, and celebrations of life services. Naturally, it is safe to share that each one had its different responses to death. The responses to their passings have ranged from relief because the loved one was suffering, to shock, because they had died without making amends with the departed, to an empty void left because the individual(s) who survived relied too much on the departed, to total confusion. Some questioned the afterlife and its possible existence. Others were concerned about how they would continue after the passing because the departed were their "soulmates" and they didn't look for love beyond the departed. All is understandable, yet what answers remain? Many.

I say this knowing fully the different avenues that one can utilize if they are willing to be open to these possibilities:

Knowing the origin of *Unlossable Love*—The very first place to find this love, as stated throughout this book, is God. He and He alone is the Author and purest form of agape/*Unlossable Love*. God has always been and will continue to always be: meaning God is forever the unstoppable source of this love. When all else seems to end or destroy this love from people in our lives, God's ability to continue throughout eternity ensures us to forever have an endless supply of agape/*Unlossable Love*. Each of us can remember a failed love in our lives and we might even have been the creator of that loss toward others. For whatever

Unlossable Love

reason, the love ended, and us/others have had our worlds rocked by the sudden loss.

If this love is found in others and not God, then we assume that this love ends when we lose contact or connection with that individual. If this is true, how can it be *Unlossable Love*?

> "No, in all these things we are more than conquerors through him who loved us. For I am sure that neither death nor life, nor angels nor rulers, nor things present nor things to come, nor powers, nor height nor depth, nor anything else in all creation, will be able to separate us from the love of God in Christ Jesus our Lord." (Romans 8:37–39)

This is what happens to each of us; believers and non-believers alike when God loves us. As we share this same form of love with others and if we are modeling it from God, we can expect this same result as we impart this love towards others; and if we are receiving this love from others, we can receive this same result. This means that this love will never be rescinded, ended, exchanged, or anything else we try to rationalize in our hearts and minds.

Allowing ourselves to love ourselves with *Unlossable Love*—As we talked about in earlier chapters, this is probably the most difficult person to love: ourselves. We are our own worst enemies because we know our own sins in the motives behind them. We can recall many, if not all of our poor choices and decisions that we have made and we carry that guilt and shame of performing such acts that have affected ourselves and others negatively. Along with all the other factors that we discussed previously, it is important to remember to allow ourselves to love one another with this *Unlossable Love* that God has shared with us and has modeled for us. Even though we may be masters of being able to share this love for others, if we do not offer this to ourselves, we are placing stipulations upon this love that should never be placed. Others will watch our lives to see if we are truly living out what we are teaching and believing. If we are not, it will be self-evident to all around us.

We have experienced firsthand what *Unlossable Love* can do for the restoration of an individual because we received this from God. If we model to others that it's okay to use this love for everyone else except ourselves, we grant them permission to do the same. Like it or not, whether you know it or not, we are all role models to someone. People will look to us for guidance and leadership. If they believe in us, they will follow our examples. If our example is for us to be able to give love to everybody else except ourselves, they too will justify in their own hearts and minds that they must do the same because that is what we are teaching them. It may not be what we intend to do, but it is the reality of our actions. Along with this, why do we want to deprive ourselves of the intimacy and blessings that we receive from *Unlossable Love* when it is something that we strive for in all of our lives with all of our relationships?

Being a father of three and a grandfather of eight children, I'm constantly under surveillance on how I respond to the various things in life. Relationships are probably the most important thing for a parent to show: relationships with our spouses, our own parents, our children/grandchildren, our friends, our peers, our coworkers, and total strangers are modeled out in front of those to whom we relate. From our examples, these individuals discovered solutions on how to react and interact with others. And these individuals will test this against social norms, faith-based theologies, the examples of others that they look up to, and of course, professionals in the field. This does not guarantee success if we are successful in our relationships with *Unlossable Love* (review the chapter that talks about running away from this love), what this does mean is that as we model this love for everyone and when we stumble, our response to that stumbling becomes a teachable moment on proper ways to move forward, stay in place, or fall back; dependent upon our response to the circumstance.

If we truly love ourselves with this love, we can provide the foundations and the roots for individuals to be able to develop positive and healthy relationships with others and to have proper self-esteem and value.

Carrying on the legacy of *Unlossable Love for others*—When our source for *Unlossable Love* dies or moves on, what happens next? That is up to us. Our response creates the next chapters of our lives. It is my hope that we focus on the positive aspect rather than the negative. How the love "ended" has a vast impact on how we move on. If the individual dies, although the act of dying is a great loss, it was ended not because of what we might have or have not done to cause the loss. Any other way of "losing" *Unlossable Love* (or the perception of the loss) causes us to blame ourselves for the loss; at least in most cases I have worked with.

I have worked at numerous places in my lifetime and have developed intimate relationships with others, both males and females. Across the board, these individuals have told me, "We'll keep in touch, I promise!" Many did for several weeks after parting ways. Others lasted a month or so. A few lasted 6 months. None lasted beyond 9 months; apart from two of my friends. It wasn't because I didn't try to reach out and try to call or meet with them. Life just happened.

At first, I thought it might have been something I had done or didn't do for the individuals. I even thought that maybe their relationship with me was one-sided: I invested more into the relationship and the others took advantage of this. This may or may not be the case, yet it was my perception. This contributed to my poor self-esteem. It wasn't until I began my work in the pastorate and mental health fields that I gained the understanding that just because we have limited contact with the individual(s) doesn't mean the love has ended; it simply means time schedules are busy with other aspects of life. As is the case with my friend Paul, each time we meet up, we pick up where we left off. The love and brotherhood we have keep going because the love *never stopped*.

Getting back to this, if someone has shown us this *Unlossable Love*, and we appreciate this love being shared with us, we can now carry the torch and pass it on to others. I look at this as a beautiful honor and privilege to do; it's a living testimony to the life which someone has provided for me and my family. Not only this, but as I long to do God's will with *Unlossable Love* for others, I find humble servanthood that God could use someone like me to make a difference in the lives of others. (This isn't a self-put down; it is acknowledging how God can use anyone at any time for every purpose that brings glory and restoration.) As I live this out, I praise God for those individuals who have invested in me and passed on what they have done or currently are doing for me. It is my prayer that others might do the same in my honor someday.

Understand we can't force someone to love us or accept our *Unlossable Love*—Remember that love never forces itself on others. We can love in the same manner as God loves us: He presents us His agape/*Unlossable Love* and it's there for whenever we need it or want it. A gift isn't a gift until we accept it. Our love is that gift. The people know how I accept their gift by whether or not I utilize their gift. Love is the ONLY gift you can regift and keep at the same time! God gives of Himself in His love and remains that Love. When we reflect on this attitude in our lives, God empowers us to have the same ability as He does. It doesn't matter if the person doesn't love us back in the same manner as we do them. A good example of this is found in the book of John:

> *"When they had finished breakfast, Jesus said to Simon Peter, "Simon, son of John, do you love me more than these?" He said to him, "Yes, Lord; you know that I love you." He said to him,*

Unlossable Love

> *"Feed my lambs." He said to him a second time, "Simon, son of John, do you love me?" He said to him, "Yes, Lord; you know that I love you." He said to him, "Tend my sheep." He said to him the third time, "Simon, son of John, do you love me?" Peter was grieved because he said to him the third time, "Do you love me?" and he said to him, "Lord, you know everything; you know that I love you." Jesus said to him, "Feed my sheep. Truly, truly, I say to you, when you were young, you used to dress yourself and walk wherever you wanted, but when you are old, you will stretch out your hands, and another will dress you and carry you where you do not want to go." (This he said to show by what kind of death he was to glorify God.) And after saying this he said to him, "Follow me." (John 21:15–19)*

This passage takes place after Peter's denial of three times of knowing Jesus Christ. He had gone off and wept bitterly after realizing what he had done to his Lord and Savior. Jesus had been crucified, buried, and risen from the dead at this point. Jesus had appeared to the Disciples several times prior to this meeting. Jesus was about to ascend into heaven to be reunited with God the Father. Unknown to Peter; Jesus was about to present the greatest example of *Unlossable Love* ever recorded in the Scriptures.

Jesus asks Peter, *". . . Do you love Me?"* Many commentaries share that the first two times Jesus asks this of Paul, His question was focused on *agape* love. The last time Peter is asked this by Jesus, the commentaries show a change from *agape* love to *phileo* (brotherly/friendship) love. This doesn't mean that Peter loved Jesus any less; it simply means at that moment Peter's understanding of the question Jesus presented registered with him. Maybe it was because Peter felt guilty for denying Jesus and was struggling with forgiving himself (I believe this to be the case). Jesus points out that He knows the depths of Peter's love by his knowledge of the way Peter would one day be martyred. At the same time, Jesus allows Peter to love him in the manner he could at the time and didn't force the issues.

In the same way, as we allow others the same graces which Jesus offers Peter, we will find that allowing others to accept our love and give their love towards us at their pace, will mature in healthy manners and have stronger roots. This is also a sign that shows patience, which is needed to develop the ability to accept the love given. As stated earlier, we sometimes struggle with accepting love because real love is foreign to so many of us.

Realizing our *Unlossable Love* comes from various sources— Probably the most noticeable and painful aspect of losing our source of *Unlossable Love* is the fear that the love ends. It will feel this is a solid truth; however, it's the farthest thing from the truth.

I know several people who believe that if *only* this person loves me, I have it all. Wrong. This might be something we try to convince ourselves of, but it's very unrealistic. God created us to be relational. This means that we are unhappy unless we have multiple relationships to draw from.

I truly love my wife with all that I am, and I cherish every moment spent with her. However, there are plenty of times she needs a break from me! Again, this isn't a put-down but a realization that there is more to her life than just me. Putting God's relationship aside for the moment, my wife has needs that I can't (no matter how *awesome* of a husband I am) meet. We are multi-relational because we are created this way.

Because God is the Author of our love, He knows our every need. He then takes these needs and provides for these same needs. I know that I need multiple relationships to complete my needs and for me to complete their needs. It's mutual and effective for having complete love and self-worth. Their love compliments my love and helps me to mature. My love does the same for those who accept my love. I get my cup filled with several different resources. Because of this, even though I would miss the departed one, there are more resources available to me. *This doesn't discount the one who passed or left!* The one who died or left is a part of the countless and endless abundance, which God provides through Himself and others. Some might ask if this is like when a pet dies, do we go right out and replace it with a different pet? Not the same thing. We can't replace the love given to us; we cherish it and count ourselves blessed to have been part of their love.

Death doesn't end our *Unlossable Love*; it strengthens it—Discovered earlier in our book, the Scriptures tells us that *nothing* can separate us from the love of God; including death. Jesus defeated death once and for all, making His Love matchless to none other. At the same time, He also empowers us to have the same ability to love others in this same manner.

It has been 18 years since my granddaughters Rebecca and Stephanie died. My mother passed away 25 years ago. My father died 6 years ago. My father-in-law died earlier this year. Did I stop loving them? Not on your life! My love continues to grow every day for them. Not only because of my faith in God and the resurrection of Christ that I know I will be reunited with these loved ones; but because I have noted that my accounts of the wrongs they might have done or perceived to have done are harder to recall and all the ways they blessed and enriched my life comes to mind more clearly and causes me great joy to have been a part of their blessing to the world. Death only removes the physical body from us. The memories, the joys, the spirit, and the heart of the loved ones remain.

Should we dwell on our loss more than the joy of having been part of the blessings of *Unlossable Love*. If this is our focus, we will lose everything: hope, the blessing of the love planted within us, the ability to move forward and being used by God for whatever purpose He calls us to. Our grief will consume us and cause us to become stagnant in our other relationships with others. It might cause us anger and rage; especially if someone else was the cause of our loved one's death (acts of

When Our Source of Unlossable Love Dies—The Impact

violence towards the loved one, maybe an accidental death, etc . . .). We can and often do seclude ourselves and withdraw from relationships when we focus mainly on our loss.

It doesn't stop there, . . . As the pain and memories haunt us and we try to escape, we might attempt to lose ourselves in different vices, such as substances, rage, anger, risky behaviors (driving too fast, taking chances which could cause harm or death to self and others), seeking revenge in the form of justice, develop suicidal ideations and/or attempt of suicide, and even suicide completion. Our happiness no longer exists. Nothing has meaning to us because the pain is too great, and we don't have the tools or the abilities to reach out for help because we believe we are totally alone in this dark world. We turn out the lights and wander in the darkness of the shadows of our souls.

Sound scary? Hopeless? It should. That darkness that we attempt to hide in turns into the tomb in which we die in; unless someone comes and breathes the breath of Life within us. If we are in this place, we can't experience the resurrection of our souls because we have forbidden our risen Savior to enter. It doesn't mean we have to *remain* in this self-imposed hell because God's love is ever-present and awaiting our call to come and save us. The true question is: Can we remember this during our sufferings and loss?

There are many other impacts that we can discuss and debate on this topic. The truth is that we can choose to focus on whatever we want. No one knows better about loss than a man from the Old Testament—Job:

> *"Now there was a day when his sons and daughters were eating and drinking wine in their oldest brother's house, and there came a messenger to Job and said, "The oxen were plowing and the donkeys feeding beside them, and the Sabeans fell upon them and took them and struck down the servants with the edge of the sword, and I alone*

have escaped to tell you." While he was yet speaking, there came another and said, "The fire of God fell from heaven and burned up the sheep and the servants and consumed them, and I alone have escaped to tell you." While he was yet speaking, there came another and said, "The Chaldeans formed three groups and made a raid on the camels and took them and struck down the servants with the edge of the sword, and I alone have escaped to tell you." While he was yet speaking, there came another and said, "Your sons and daughters were eating and drinking wine in their oldest brother's house, and behold, a great wind came across the wilderness and struck the four corners of the house, and it fell upon the young people, and they are dead, and I alone have escaped to tell you."

*Then **Job** arose and tore his robe and shaved his head and fell on the ground and worshipped. And he said, "Naked I came from my mother's womb, and naked shall I return. The Lord gave, and the Lord has taken away; blessed be the name of the Lord." (Job 1:13–21)*

The story of Job is present in the Old Testament and God gives us great insight into what was taking place at that time. There are those who are nonbelievers who would read this book of Job and talk about how evil God is to allow an innocent man like Job to go through all that he did as recorded in the book. Not that I must defend God; God is not the Author of the events but allow these events to take place to survive for a far greater purpose than what we can understand in our finite minds. Still, there are people who would still believe God is evil for allowing it to happen.

In this story, Satan comes to God and states that he (Satan) can cause Job to turn away from God and curse Him. Thus, Satan removes everything from Job; apart from a wife who kept nagging him to curse God and die and friends who believe that Job must've done something extremely wrong for God's wrath the fall upon him the way that they believed it to be. As you continue to read the story, we take note of God's agape/*Unlossable Love* being ever-present as evidenced by God's protection over Job's life and the final blessing that Job receives at the end of the book. (I would encourage each of you to read this on your own as time presents itself to you.)

If ever man had a reason to put himself in a dark place and to seclude himself for the rest of his life, Job would be that man! However, as we see in the passage provided, Job continually praises the Lord and remembers how much his God loves him and has provided for him (and will continue to do so). Job had every reason to focus on the darkness yet continued to remember the love of God. THAT led him to remain hopeful and content.

If you are currently going through tough times, have lost a loved one who is or was your source of *Unlossable Love,* and feel as if you're all alone; you're not. God is with you, and He has provided people to love you through your pain and sorrows. Don't allow the darkness to overcome you and imprison your soul or spirit. Count the blessings of those who have died and have presented you with *Unlossable Love.*

CARRYING ON WITH UNLOSSABLE LOVE

There's a movie from 2000 called *Pay It Forward*, in which a young boy named Trevor McKinney (played by Haley Joel Osment) has a class assignment in which he tries to prove that if someone does something kind for someone else and instead of receiving a reward or payment for this task, he instructs the person he helped to "pay it forward" doing something nice for someone else, a cycle begins. Trevor thought that if everyone would do this, the world might become a better place.

Based on a true story, Trevor's idea had, at first, its many struggles. Yet, Trevor persevered in his quest and literally gave his life in making this movement come true; at least for one young boy, he was protected from being bullied. Trevor's death is a testimony to God inspiring one person to make a difference. It didn't have to be on a grand scale (which this did for his town and eventually the movie which made it worldwide), but even if that one person he helped helps someone else and they pass it on, the world becomes a better place for all. I weep every time I watch or even think about it because the impact it has on me motivates me to "pay it forward".

Looking at my life and the many different experiences which could have made me quite different as a person if those people whom God provided to help me weren't there for me, I see and feel the desperate necessity for "paying it forward" to all who would like to take advantage of the opportunities. Not boasting except in the Lord; I have done this and continue to mentor, encourage, and empower anyone whom God brings into my life.

In some instances, our time is short but impactful for all involved. In other cases, it continues to be slower and more paced with God's timing. In all cases, I share what I have been mentored, love as I have been loved, discipline as I was disciplined and encourage each to add their heart's calling to what they have learned. As I did this, they mentored me with their wisdom and knowledge; helping me to reach those who are younger. They assisted me in connecting to their generation in a way they would accept me and what I must share. *Unlossable Love* works this way!

Just because we finally have received the *Unlossable Love* we have sought for all our lives doesn't give us a reason to cease our search for or acceptance of this love. *It is the beginning of our task!* This love that we now possess demands perseverance and commitment from us. We can't simply sit back and bask in love; love demands movement and a constant flow. A river has a constant flow to it. People have tried to tame the river and change its course; however, the river continues to flow. That consistency in that strength to persevere allows the river to be what it is. Likewise, *Unlossable Love* enables us and empowers us to be what we are in the eyes of God and even in the eyes of others.

I am one of the fortunate souls who were able to receive this love (even though I did not know what it was called at the time, I still see that it truly is God's agape/*Unlossable Love*) at a young age and how it helped me to become the person that I am today. And even though I see evidence of this love in my life in many different areas, my soul continually craves more of this love in all aspects of my life. Because of the overflow of this love, I am able to share and mentor others into receiving this and sharing this with others. God gives me all the opportunities to "pay it forward" with the hopes that lives are changed and blessed by my efforts.

I do this not because of vanity or self-glorification, like the woman at the well story found in John chapter 4, I tell others because of the way that I've been blessed and healed from this. All glory goes to God; for he is the Author of the *Unlossable Love* which I now have. I am humbled to share this gift with others and have the pleasure of seeing lives changed. You can experience this as well when you develop this love in your life. Like that river, it will flow out of you and flow naturally into your community; supplying this community with the resources it needs to thrive in compassion and grace.

If you are like me, you may start off feeling that the sharing of this *Unlossable Love* might feel like an obligation: since it was this love that saved me, I felt that it was my duty to pass it on to others. All my passion was not in it at the beginning. This is a natural feeling and feeling that you should address. Obviously, we are not "obligated" or feel that we have a sense of duty to share this with others because we are just learning about *Unlossable Love* and all that it is. Besides, you can't share what you don't know. As his love became more apparent to me and I began to heal because of its presence in my life, it was my joy that motivated me to share with those that I know and/or assumed were struggling in the same manner that I was. Joy motivated me to share in my thankfulness towards God and others and empowered me to persevere. Are we called to love others? Absolutely yes! Do we desire to love others? Again, absolutely yes! Then it should become natural for us to share *Unlossable Love* as we become comfortable with it and become experts in this love.

Carrying on with *Unlossable Love* in both our personal lives and the lives we invest in, I believe, is the greatest form of worship to God. The Disciples understood that Jesus' way of ministry vastly differed from the Proper Church with its traditions and rituals. There was too much legalism taking place and many of the religious leaders lost sight of their callings to serve God's people and their communities. They taught *religion* and Jesus taught *relationships*. There truly is a great difference between the two and the responses are proof of this truth. People come to Jesus Christ because they see genuine love coming from Him (the agape/*Unlossable*

Love) and receive instant acceptance without any obligations or demands from Him. Even if someone wants to argue that when Jesus commands us to stop a certain behavior or attitude, He does this to assist our healing and turn away from the very things which caused the inflictions we have. The choice remains ours and so do the natural and spiritual responses to our actions that come with the decisions we make. God informs us so we can make informed decisions as to what we desire and pursue.

> ***Beloved**, let us love one another, for love is from God, and whoever loves has been born of God and knows God. Anyone who does not love does not know God, because God is love. In this the love of God was made manifest among us, that God sent his only Son into the world, so that we might live through him. In this is love, not that we have loved God but that he loved us and sent his Son to be the propitiation for our sins. Beloved, if God so loved us, we also ought to love one another. No one has ever seen God; if we love one another, God abides in us and his love is perfected in us.*
>
> *By this we know that we abide in him and he in us, because he has given us of his Spirit. And we have seen and testify that the Father has sent his Son to be the Savior of the world. Whoever confesses that Jesus is the Son of God, God abides in him, and he in God. So we have come to know and to believe the love that God has for us. God is love, and whoever abides in love abides in God, and God abides in him. By this is love perfected with us, so that we may have confidence for the Day of Judgment, because as he is so also are we in this world. There is no fear in love, but perfect love casts out fear. For fear has to do with punishment, and whoever fears has not been perfected in love. We love because he first loved us. If anyone says, "I love God," and hates his brother, he is a liar; for he who does not love his brother whom he has seen cannot love God whom he has not seen. And this commandment*

> *we have from him: whoever loves God must also love his brother.*
> *(1 John 4:7–21)*

I share this passage to share what the Scriptures ask us as believers to follow. The passage isn't asking us to do anything that He (God/Christ/Holy Spirit) hasn't already done for each of us. This is how God sees how we mirror His love towards Him as we mirror it toward others. This is an evidence-based practice that has noticeable and measurable results and outcomes. As we continue with the *Unlossable Love* bestowed to us, others are drawn to this love and desire its healing powers.

People want to change for the better. I believe this is a fact. Yet, circumstances, negative influences, generational differences, social norms which differ from each generation, traumas, and low or no self-worth impair some to have neither the ability nor the desire to change. Some believe this is "just the way life is and will be for me. . . . " If this is the way you think and believe, it could very much be this for you.

However, this isn't what God wants for us and He is doing all He can to show us that we are better than this by being in our life. People accept this thought process because they're uninformed about the ability to have a choice. Even if they know they have a choice, many don't have the strength or the support to follow through with their desire to change. As we carry on with *Unlossable Love*, we become those supports for others.

When these individuals begin to gain their strength in this love, they become more independent and pass on this love to those they connect with. This breaks the generational curse which prevents families from breaking unhealthy cycles and lifestyles by showing the options available to break away.

Beatrice and I encourage you, the reader, to consider all that you've read in this book and to listen to God's voice for you. Maybe He is calling you to His agape/*Unlossable Love* and trying to bring healing to you and yours. It's possible that He is calling you to extend this love to others. It could also be to make us aware of the pain and brokenness which we or others try to deal with alone and in seclusion of the support available to them. You might be called to serve like Beatrice and Kenneth in foster care, like me in a form of ministry/outreach, or whatever God places on your hearts. And, just maybe, God is showing you how you already have identified His agape/*Unlossable Love* in your life and to show you how He has and always will be present in your life. Whatever the case might be, we pray that this book helps you to reach your fullest potential for yourself and your loved ones. May God richly bless you! Carry on with your *Unlossable Love*.

BONUS FEATURE—STORIES FROM LIVES THAT EXPERIENCED UNLOSSABLE LOVE

For this portion of the book, I am drawing from my past interactions with individuals with whom I have had the humble pleasure (and continue to have an ongoing relationship with) of utilizing *Unlossable Love* over years past. Each of the individuals comes from my involvement in three different vocations I had been a part of a juvenile center, a mental health agency, and my church setting. I had reached out to these individuals once God had placed them on my heart as I wrote this book with Beatrice. Our stories are interconnected with one another and, I believe, their transformations came about from the provisions God had for these individuals during their most important time of need.

As stated throughout this writing, I have stressed that these stories are NOT to glorify myself or Beatrice/Kenneth but to give examples of those whose lives have been transformed by God's love and the love we extend to others. All that the Fosters and I can do is solely because God has called us, empowers us, and strengthened us to achieve His will.

DAWN'S STORY

In these chapters, I asked each person a series of questions and asked them to respond to said questions. The questions are added so you can view the responses each provided in their own words. The first contributor is a young lady named Dawn. I worked with her at the juvenile center in the 1990s–2000s. She was in her young teens and had already experienced more in life than someone her age should have. I will not share details due to confidentiality aspects, yet Dawn shares her story with us. I have been connected to her since that time. In her eyes, I'm her adopted dad; a title she shares and I am humbled to be for her (and others).

- What were your thoughts about the circumstance(s) which caused you to feel the way you did when you first engaged with me? This isn't about me; it's more about you and where you were as a person at that time.

"When I first met you I was in a place where I wasn't in trouble but I was on the borderlands of crossing over to more destructive behaviors, I gravitated towards you because the other girls around me trusted you and spoke of how you really cared and listened. After I spoke with you I remember thinking I wish my dad would have spoken those words to me and listened to me the way you had, as the years passed you saw the destructiveness come out, the episodes of anger and hostility, and yet you still gave me hug and reassured me I wasn't a monster."

- What did you feel about yourself during this time(s)? Self-worth? Value to others? Peers?

I had no self-value or self-love during these times, I hid the fact that other people's opinions were important to me, to a damaging point. I felt like a feral animal caged, and I was reliving abuse and trauma I had experienced in my formation years.

- What did relationships look like then?

Relationships and how I viewed them were from a very unloving, skewed perception, the abuse I experienced in my early life that made me feel if I wasn't pleasing someone, I wasn't worthy of love. If you weren't being yelled at or beaten, you were ignored and made to feel invisible, relationships weren't meant to last, and you would always get hurt.

- What helped you to feel Unlossable Love from God, family, and/or others?

Finding out I was pregnant with my oldest daughter, realizing she would always love me. There were different moments in life when I was at a low point and I was reminded how loved and amazing I was, that I was worth digging out of that hole, that my contribution to life really mattered. It was mostly from people that weren't my blood, but my spiritually made family, their love for me brought me closer to my higher power and best self.

- What helped you to make the changes you did? What struggles did you face during your time of change? Who/what helped you to continue your changes?

My children, the friends I buried, and the mentors that guided me have been catalysts to my life changes. I faced homelessness, addiction, exploitation, and alienation from my own child. Realizing the cycle can stop with me at any time, having those constants in my life even when I wasn't constantly, gently, encouraging me to be kind to myself and that it really was okay to start over and having faith that one day it's going to get better. Becoming whole has been a practice of loving every part of myself and finding peace in knowing my children will never experience what I did.

- What does your life look like now? Are they the changes you desired?

My life now is not where I want it to be but the steps are there to get it where I want it, being sober has helped clarify those steps, and working hard every day to make my dreams come true. I've made some beautiful changes that have helped, so many, and it keeps me inspired to create those beautiful changes for myself. I would say intrinsically it's everything I've desired. My self-love is infinite and I'm no longer ashamed of my past.

- What advice would you give to others?

My best advice is some of us go through things unimaginable to be a voice for the voiceless, and as much as we get in our own way, we are the ones who got us this far, no one else made us get out of bed and make the best of each day, we do that, and we're worth it, you can truly create whatever you put your mind to, just never give up or stop believing in a better day.

- Talk about how your life was when we first met. You can go as deep as you want her as light as you want, and you can change names if you would like as well.

When I first met you I was a child of chaos and pain, I was just acknowledging the abuse I had experienced growing up and I didn't react well to feeling so used and disposable. I had just met my mom and partying like I was grown at 13, my mom was just discovering the abuse I went through and we didn't have the resources or support to navigate these things alone. My actions led to me being institutionalized and later placed in foster care. By the time I graduated high school I had attended 23 schools across 2 states, I lost count of the places I lived, and looked for love in all the wrong places.

- If you've ever felt unlovable or like an outcast, please talk about those feelings. What were the things that helped you to see beyond the negativity to see your potential in the eyes of God, yourself, your community, and so on…?

I struggled with feeling accepted for a long time and was bullied until I was 13. My interpretation of a parent was one who was absent, abusive, critical, and cold, friends weren't really friends, and I weaponized my abuse by dating older men, thinking they would "take care of me" when in all reality I was just a mule and an object of their satisfaction. My pain and sadness turned to rage, I was out of control, attempted suicide twice, and had no respect for authority. Honestly meeting you taught me who God really was, you were the only male figure I had growing up that was kind and caring. You helped me open my heart up to see I wasn't what I had been shown most of my life. When I graduated high school and went on to be an advocate, I realized so many others had stories like mine and it made me feel like I belonged, that my will to live and love defied the abuse and generational cycle that was set before me and I really was a key to changing that cycle for my children. As I came into adulthood, still struggling with addiction, I continued to do social work that helped others, realizing we're human with human conditioning, giving space to love those who otherwise didn't love themselves. Now being sober and in my 30s I look back and realize the more I shared my story and helped others the more it has healed me and made me whole.

- Please share your experiences with those you have helped and used Unlossable Love with and the impacts it had.

Some people I have helped, and they've continued down a destructive path, but they know I always have love and encouragement for them, some have come into adulthood and made something of themselves being inspired by my work and life story, and some have passed on but I carry their stories with me so their children have a better understanding when they come of age and have questions. I feel my love for others created a ripple, and no matter the outcome, impacted them for the better, I've seen the work I started 14 years ago come full circle 3 times now through some of the students and youth I mentored and I'm humbled that I planted those seeds seeing how they nurtured and grew them.

As you can see, Dawn has overcome some incredible obstacles in her lifetime. She could have easily become a statistic where her past traumas and experiences, along with poor choices could have made her remain in the dark shadows she was once overcome by. Because of various people, God, and the knowledge that she was and remains precious to

God and others. Dawn spoke about the various battles she faced with self-worth, trust and faith issues, irrational thought processes and misconceptions, and facing her own demons. I know from working with her the times when she struggled, when she fought against assistance, the accountability on her behalf, and mine as well. As she pointed out so well, it wasn't anyone else who could claim her success; she alone did the work necessary to overcome her past and change her future. Dawn also proves my point of how *Unlossable Love*, once understood, becomes a passion for us to share with others.

Even though Dawn has come a long way in her growth, she continues to deal with past issues and struggles from time to time. She is a work in progress. All of us are like Dawn in the fact that we are all works in progress. This shows the importance of the necessity of being consistent with *Unlossable Love*. Dawn also remembers that as she gives this love to others, she must be able to accept it for herself. There is no exact amount of time that a person can be designated for healing and restoration. We are all different, respond differently, and heal differently. Based on how much baggage we carry with us in our lives, some will heal quickly while others take a lifetime. A person's fortitude establishes the pace in how one responds to *Unlossable Love* given to us by God and one another.

Because of knowing Dawn in the ways that I do, I can share that she has overcome a great deal throughout her life; even more than what she has shared. Many of us do not like to talk about the trials and tribulations that we've gone through and their impacts on us because it feels like when we do, it's like taking a scab off a very deep wound: the moment we rip it open, the wound is exposed, the pain becomes more intense, and we are not sure if we could ever heal from it. Many of the dark places that Dawn had visited in her journey made her blind to the possibilities that lay within her. It took a matter of time before Dawn was able to realize that she was a victim of many of the things that she went through.

At the same time, the influences of those experiences also caused her to go into dark places of her own. Whether it be for escaping the pain, seeking revenge and justice, or hearing people say that these things would help her; only to find out that they ended her and sometimes destroyed her in the midst of it, only Dawn and God know what brought her to those places. The one thing that I do know, and Dawn knows this now as well, is that it was God in his agape/*Unlossable Love* that has restored her thus far and will continue to restore her until her completion.

JUSTIN'S STORY

Another individual I have the pleasure of not only mentoring and helping to know and understand what *Unlossable Love* is but also call him my "adopted" son is Justin. I am humbled to call him a friend and "spiritual son"; one whom I continue to mentor. We met shortly after I became a pastor for Pleasant Lake United Methodist Church (PLUM as we call it). This took place in the early 2000s when Justin and I met. There was something about him that God put on my heart to take him under my wing and simply love and care for him. As you read Justin's responses to his questions, try to look at the various struggles which he shares. His vulnerability here is of great importance for a wide audience…

- What were your thoughts about the circumstance(s) which caused you to feel the way you did when you first engaged with me? This isn't about me; it's more about you and where you were as a person at that time.

   I met you, John, at a time when I was wrestling with a lot of different adversities, which raised many questions in my life. A couple of those questions were the following:
   "What does it mean to be a great man?"
   "Where does my identity lie?"
   "Can I trust someone other than myself?"
   "Will I always feel like I am fighting these battles alone?"

Justin's Story

You and I began our relationship in the midst of some of the hardest realities I have faced in my life. The first one was the discovery of my father's infidelity and unfaithfulness to my mom which I witnessed with my own eyes. This then resulted in the second harsh reality of my mom retreating to a season of spite and solitude which took my family out of the church. The third one is that my mom had more to worry about than "God's love." She needed to find a way to raise 4 children by herself with (at the time) zero support or help from others. What was left from middle school through high school was a household of hopelessness filled with much emotional and physical spite.

While my mother and siblings wanted nothing to do with a relationship with God (at the time), I felt a pull toward finding a place where I could seek peace. This led to me going with my friend Darius and his family to PLUM where I met you PJ (Pastor John).

Witnessing God speak through you kept my attention. And even though I was only 11-12 years old, I sat on every word that came from your sermons. But what was really the catalyst to our relationship, was the fact that you noticed my intrigue and acknowledged my excitement for God and His word.

It was the nudge of encouragement from you, that I had a purpose to do great things for His kingdom that gave me permission to lean on others. While I had that permission it didn't make it easier to submit to help, which I think is why I kept coming back to you. It was the beginning of a relationship that would help fill and sustain me even to this present day.

- What did you feel about yourself during this time(s)? Self-worth? Value to others? Peers?

At the time, I was still a kid, but I questioned my own purpose and identity every day. I desired a connection. I wanted to be acknowledged for my worth. I was bitter towards my family and used that as motivation to be great in all that I did. But it wasn't because I thought I was great; it was only to simply spite my parents who I felt betrayed me. My dad crushed the family dynamics with adultery and alcoholism, and my mom was constantly working, but when I was acknowledged, I was met with glances of disdain due to my similar appearance to my father. She never really admitted it, but I could tell I reminded her of him on a daily basis and it led to a lot of her emotions toward him being projected onto me.

To top it off, living in a community where most of the demographic doesn't look like you made me feel like an outcast. Even when I would spend the weekends with my black relatives, they looked at me the same way the white folks in my hometown did. To cope I would assimilate the mentality of whatever was most relevant to the culture and environment I was in. Similar to the abilities of a chameleon. This was my camouflage and I found more people accepted me in this manner. At the end of the day, it made me feel like an imposter and is something I fight against now in adulthood.

- What did relationships look like then?

The one consistent relationship I had from pre-teen adolescence to now has been you, PJ, and God. I have always felt I could speak out all of my frustration with God. I can rejoice with Him. I can cry with Him. I can laugh with Him. I can joke with Him. He receives me for who I am and He placed me in life so I can not only experience Him spiritually but also know that there are people here on Earth for me physically to walk with me when I need them.

I was always gifted in sports and was in all the honor classes which helped me have a lot of "friends", but you and Darius were the only ones growing whom I felt I could have solid intentional conversations."

- What helped you to feel Unlossable Love from God, family, and/or others?

"You for starters. Journaling and finding any way to record my days helped me as well. Whenever I had a bad day or a good day, I would take inventory of what I did and if I brought God into everything, I did that day and what elements in my day were aids from God.

It was no coincidence that when I recognized God's Unlossable Love in my situations I felt highly favored, and acknowledged and things went well for me. This doesn't mean I still didn't have bad days. I did, but the feeling of Peace was there which turned trials into lessons that shaped instead of scars that would never heal.

I recognized that He put you in my life as a mentor spiritually and to help me experience Him more. He placed my basketball coach and baseball coach to help build my ability to lead in capacities where God was not always felt. He also gave me other men in my life throughout college to show me that God truly is in everything we do if we acknowledge Him."

- What helped you to make the changes you made? What struggles did you face?

"You, along with my creative writing teacher in 8th Grade (Mr. Kennedy), encouraged me to start journaling. Journaling helped me express my feelings, goals, current experiences, and future aspirations on paper which resulted in me creating a process to help me make sense of my feelings and move toward my personal goals.

My journal helped me then to pray for these people, places, and things I wrote down. Prayer invited the Holy Spirit to surface in my heart more and more as I got older. I started seeing God in more of my daily life. I started reading the Bible more and setting time aside for stillness with God. The time of stillness began to soften my heart more and more each year (still have more softening to do), which has opened my eyes to the callings the Lord has encouraged me to do.

I continued to struggle with life at home. I saw zero change in my father and the only real change I saw in my mother was that she quit smoking. We were still living on a low income which made it hard to even think about having a better life for myself at times when all I was witnessing in my household was my mom stressing out about bills and debt each month.

My popularity at school continued to grow, but I was met with a lot of scrutiny because of my love for people. Some people saw me as two-faced because of the different groups at school I would associate with. I didn't care about where you came from or how popular you were. I simply enjoyed connecting so that made me appear at times shallow to some while empathetic and kind to others. I also expressed my faith outwardly which made most identify me as the "religious kid". This one always irritated me because I cared more about my relationship with God than any "religion" and always felt others were judging me based on their negative interactions with the church.

I had to fight off lies about who I was and focus more on Whose I was. I went to a school where I would experience racially insensitive jokes on a weekly basis. Whether it was teachers making comments about "the way I talk" to more intense offenses such as being called racial slurs. These challenges have only helped mold the person I am today. Being of mixed races is less of a focus of mine now because my identity is in Jesus and not in a culture, ethnicity, or skin tone.

- What helped you to make the changes you made? What struggles did you face during your time of change? Who/what helped you to continue your changes?

Staying close to those whom I felt spiritually filled me was a big key to continuing my spiritual transformation. Our youth group was small, but super intentional, which I believe was like that for a reason. I also believe keeping myself in sports and extracurriculars helped grow my love for personal development.

If I wasn't at school, in sports, or working my time was spent on things that brought me life. Having the opportunity to spend a lot of my upbringing in the church and under your mentorship shaped my mindset and gave me permission to dream bigger than the confines of my own mind.

Also, being placed in roles of leadership both in the church and out helped encourage me to keep going! It held me accountable to stay the course because I knew if I had a vision or goal to do it God would find a way and place the right people in my life. He did that with you PJ when I expressed my desire to pastor a church one day!

- What does your life look like now? Are they the changes you desired?

God is not playing checkers. He plays chess. And His tactics of choice is what you call this Unlossable Love. Looking at my life and where I am now, I know it was God. The struggles that I experienced as a young child helped equip me with what I am doing now. And that is guiding the next generation as the Youth and Young Adults Pastor at City Church Fort Wayne, Ind.

There were changes that I desired and changes that I didn't know I needed, but regardless, the change that was made has brought me, is bringing, and will continue to bring me to the goals I have in my life. One thing God is great at is preparation. He is not done with me. I feel there is more He will call on me to do from Him and I have confidence that the trials I am overcoming today will be for His will and will fulfill my purpose soon enough. My cup continues to be filled with the goals I dreamt of when I was a kid.

- What advice would you give to others?

"God's Unlossable Love will prepare you, equip you, and will always be available to you. He loves us so much that He will wait for us to come to receive that Love, but even though He waits that doesn't mean He won't nudge us or place people in our lives to help get us there.

I encourage those who are struggling to lean into challenges. Don't shy away from them and do what's easy. When we do what's easy, it's usually a temporary escape. When we lean into our trials, that is when I feel God really works to reveal the things, He has placed in our lives to conquer them. Through victory we find ever-lasting peace, knowledge to help others dealing with the same circumstances, and that Unlossable Love you have been talking about."

- Talk about how your life was when we first met. You can go as deep as you want her as light as you want, and you can change names if you would like as well.

I think my answer to question one has a nice summary of this. It was hard. I was entering a season where a lot of child trauma began. It wasn't really until I got into my serious relationship with Loren (my wife) that I truly began to acknowledge and unpack the difficulties I was wrestling with. A couple of days ago, I went back and read through some entries in my first journal and all I saw in the words were a sad young boy looking for acknowledgment, looking for love, and looking for a relationship. The one cool thing though, was that at the end of almost all the entries I wrote in my journals, I finish with a prayer, a Bible verse, a truth from God, and sign my signature at the bottom.

I never understood why I started doing that, but it is something I still do. I think it's because no matter what kind of day I am having be it a good one or bad one, I have always felt (even during my hard days as a kid) the presence of God's Unlossable Love. And I needed to finish every day pointing my direction back to God and my signature was the stamping of that commitment.

- If you've ever felt unlovable or like an outcast talk about those feelings. What were the things that helped you to see beyond the negativity to see your potential in the eyes of God, yourself, your community, and so on?

God's people are very messy. We see that throughout the Bible and within our congregations and I am not an exception. I make mistakes. I have muddied the waters and I have overstepped boundaries that have resulted in me losing touch with close family, friends, and church members. I am a harsh critic of myself to the point where I fall prey to old lies, I believed in myself when I was young, "Your stupid. You mess everything up. You're an imposter. You aren't making a difference. You do more damage than good.

During those moments, what helps the most is to be around people who love me. If I can't surround myself with those people, I go to the Scriptures and read what God has to say about me. I pray to Him and tell Him my feelings and surrender to His will and ask for Peace. I also look back to where I started and notice all the progress I have made because of His love and direction.

- Your experiences with those you have helped and used Unlossable Love with and the impacts it had.

Because of God's Unlossable Love, I've had the privilege to help other young kids some of whom are now young adults know God's Unlossable Love and I continue to do so full-time within the church where I now have the opportunity to minister to hundreds of students, young adults and parents on a weekly basis!

Justin and I continue in our relationship and even as I mentor him; he also mentors me in knowing how to connect with his generation and some of the more recent generations. His presence in these generations helps him to have his finger on their pulse, which they grant him entrance into their lives because they can see that he "gets them" and can connect *where they are* instead of expecting them to connect with him first. This is where God's agape/*Unlossable Love* shines its brightest.

I can see Justin becoming a life changer to those he ministers to; not because I assisted in his mentoring, but because of the heart God developed within him. It's Justin allowing God to shine in him and work through him. *Unlossable Love* helps us to *long for and desire to* have God use us to help bring healing and restore others (or even ourselves). Because of the different situations and the experiences he had faced, others who are experiencing these or who have experienced these can see how God is able to bring about change if we are open to that change. Justin was receptive; even though he was young and broke more than he knew.

KATELYN'S STORY

Katelyn and I first met when she was 14 years old. I ran a program called Moral Recognition Therapy (MRT) and Katelyn was one of my students. This program is an evidence-based practice in which we address the various things that we allow ourselves to be imprisoned by; it could be addictions, traumas, and a host of other things to name a few. Katelyn was in all forms of crisis: poor family relationships, addictions, depression, and low self-esteem. Naturally, Katelyn was overwhelmed by everything and everyone, and her behavior reflected this. Yet, I could tell that she needed someone to be there for her, no matter how hard she fought back against it.

As Katelyn engaged in the MRT program, she fought against it: she had already gone through multiple counselors and therapists (and some of this will be shared within this chapter a little later) whom she thought never really invested in *her for herself*, but only did it "because they were being paid to be there". Naturally, when a person feels this way, it's no wonder they would never invest in a program or various people who never really tries to see them for who they are and to hear their voices without judgment.

When I asked Katelyn if she would like to share her story, she was only more than happy to share this because she believes that her story could possibly help others in their walk through the struggles of their lives. Katelyn asked me to interview her and here are the results of that interview, along with the questions:

- Can you share with me what your life looked like at the time we met? You can share whatever you like.

I was a broken person. I was godless. I was addicted to pills, and I drank a lot. I had been expelled for the second time for drugs from another school and I overdosed. I woke up in the hospital the week before we had met. When I first met you, I attended a summer group for kids. I can't remember what it was called but it was before I started the MRT group. I had even come to the group drunk on my first day. I was a godless and promiscuous person at that time in my life. I was prepared to die shortly. I thought nobody or anything was going to get through to me or would be able to help me or make me want to care about my life.

- What was MRT like when you first attended? What were your thoughts about it?

I thought it was very stereotypical on my first day. I thought, like everything else in my life, I was going to be thrown into a category with other people and slip through the cracks. I was always kind of invisible to any help given to me. But I knew by day two I was completely wrong. We were each seen as an individual person who cared about our own individual needs and support. And it wasn't a shame on your group like I thought it was going to be. I had been in groups before, and it wasn't the same as the others. It was a place of forgiveness, love, and support where everyone leaned on everyone; helping each other through the things we all had going on. Whether it was drug abuse, alcohol abuse, or anger management issues, we were all seen as individuals. It was my first time experiencing it and it actually saved my life to be cared about in this way. We were not a job to you; the others and I were involved; we were a mission. I was finally seen, and I finally allowed myself the help I needed because I finally felt safe too.

- What caused you to know that you could trust after you've been through so much broken trust?

It was the non-judgment and consistent reassurance you gave us all. It was like, "We all make mistakes..." and the pep talks and how we could relapse or mess up but could never lose your respect. The only thing we ever got when we messed up was extra help and that's enough to make any hurt child trust. Instead of the shame we got from everywhere else, we had actual support from caring adults, and it made me want to try harder. It made me realize that I didn't have to give up. I just had to be honest with myself and others because I already had the help I needed.

- Did *Unlossable Love* ever exist to you? What impact does *Unlossable Love* have on your life today? Do you share this love with others?

God's Unlossable Love did. Your Unlossable Love; you loved us all like your own. Most of us didn't have parents that invested as much time into us as you had. I now share the same understanding and forgiveness and complete acceptance in the Unlossable Love I give my daughter every day in her life. I also share that Unlossable Love with God as He has me and all the rest of His children . . . another thing I learned from you. You taught me that love when you chose to see us as people with problems instead of the problems of people.

- What would you like to share with someone who is struggling, afraid of loving others/themselves, or who has lost hope?

That life is too short . . . It took me until I was 20 years to realize how fast life was going by. It goes in the blink of an eye and by the time you reach 20, you only have a few more 20s left. You have got to use every day to your advantage. Work on you for you and nobody else. You can be at your lowest and the only way you have is up. God doesn't give anyone more than they can handle ever in our lives. Everything we go through builds our character; it's not what you go through but how you get through it that shows who you ARE. If you're in a bad place, you have to be able to love yourself first before you can love anyone else. Every time you feel like it's the end, it's really just the end of a chapter and God is just opening the door to what's next. Instead of looking at it like it's a loss, take from it everything you can. Learn from the hard things and you can never lose when you're gaining experience and knowledge. He's planning your next big chapter; building moments in your life.

Katelyn and I are still connected today. We stay in contact with one another and keep each other up to date with what's going on in life. As I read the responses to Katelyn's questions, I find myself both humbled and proud: humble that God would use someone like me to have such an impact on Katelyn (I give ALL glory to God because He was the One who led me to work with Katelyn and others and proud because Katelyn is a very beautiful person both inside and out!). Katelyn shared so much of herself to help others never give up on themselves or those they love. I have always thought of Katelyn as my reason for doing what I do in life because she has shown me and taught me as much as I have hopefully taught her.

Please take to heart Katelyn's story and her words. She has been where some of you are right now. No matter how hopeless it seems to be for you, life can and does get better if you allow yourself to have faith; in God, others, and yourself.

FINAL WORDS

I want to begin these final words by giving all glory to God; this book, all of my and Beatrice's experiences (along with her family), and how we responded to their experiences are directly a result of God gifting us with the various gifts, talents, wisdom, and openness to the Holy Spirit's leading. Speaking for Beatrice and myself, we are thankful that we were privileged enough to be a part of some AMAZING lives that we have!

People often tell us, "It takes a special person to do what you do . . ." or "I could never do what you do for others; I'm not sure I could do it." Both Beatrice and I are just as ordinary as you are; the difference is that each of us knows personally how we were once like those we help, and someone had *Unlossable Love* for us as we needed it most. Someone saw potential in us, had seen the depths of brokenness we experienced, or witnessed how much we needed someone to rescue us from ourselves and our situations. We are not saints, just people used by God to bring restoration and healing to those whom God entrusts to our care. We are not perfect in *any* manner, but we are open to change and to show others how to change their stars to shine brightly and joyfully.

Unlossable Love is for *everybody!* Yes, many of those whom Beatrice and I have worked with and continue to assist our youths; however, we also work with everyone we relate to; family, coworkers, friends, strangers, different agencies, and people in the church. God hasn't given us these gifts and talents to share with selected individuals, but with all.

It is our hope that this book is a tool that empowers you, the readers, to develop *Unlossable Love* for yourself and those you relate to. Beatrice and

I are not the only ones called to this; *you are also invited* to share in this ministry. Even if you don't have a faith system like ours, *Unlossable Love* transcends all faiths, cultures, and belief systems.

As noted in Katelyn's story, people are starving for someone to see them, their struggles, and their hopelessness and to love them not because of being paid to care for them, but to honestly and whole-heartedly love without expecting anything in return. Trust us, both of us have had people reject us and our help. It was heartbreaking to see these individuals throw away their lives to the lies and heartaches they faced or are facing. We are still standing by whenever they need us. But for those who have accepted *Unlossable Love*, it's such a blessing to see lives changed forever because they finally had someone care enough for them.

You might be thinking, "But I'm not comfortable working with youth or whoever . . . " That's fine because all of us connect to different people. Let me list a few of the different people whom you might be open to working with (this is just a partial listing, but you can add more if you are so inclined):

- **Those in the judicial system**—People who have been incarcerated for whatever reason are often outcasts from society. Yes, some might be hardened, but most of these individuals have made poor choices only one time and carry a lifetime sentence of being labeled and shunned for their crimes. Too many see their past and not their potential. I personally know several individuals who have had completely positive life changes and yet still struggle with a past label given to them by society. You can assist in their acceptance by seeing them as God sees them: precious and loved. It should also be noted that this isn't just for adults, but also juveniles as well. We are seeing a rapid increase of juveniles becoming involved with delinquent acts for a number of reasons.
- **LGBTQ+**—Here is a group that has *so many* struggles, more so than the average person. Regardless of what you might think,

LGBTQ+ individuals have been shunned by society, religious organizations, *from their own families* for being who they are, and in some countries, murdered or cast into prisons. You may not have to agree with their lifestyles/choices, but you must see them deserving the same love and respect that everyone else has and expects. Substance abuses, mental illness/challenges, and suicide attempts and completions are much higher than any other group (with possibly the exception of military/veterans, which could be equal to LGBTQ+). This group experiences more hatred and judgment than most other groups. I believe you will agree that they also have God's *Unlossable Love*, but are *we* also willing to grant this same love from ourselves? If we take the time and effort, we'll soon see how much we are alike than we are different…

- **Military/veterans**—Like LGBTQ+ individuals, this group also suffers from rejection and loneliness. It was recently reported that a veteran will complete suicide 1 every 8 minutes. Many are homeless and suffer from broken relationships for numerous reasons. Chemical addictions run rampant in this group, trying to self-medicate their mental and emotional sufferings. People don't understand that these veterans *don't share or open up* to regular counselors and therapists because many are not trained for their special needs and experiences. Most veterans *will not open up* because 1) Military personnel are classified with many things and to share these, many different consequences can occur if revealed, 2) No veteran will discuss with civilian therapists/counselors because there is no possible way for these to understand the unique circumstances/situations these veterans have experienced, 3) The guilt is too great to express—in war, no one wins. Battle scars mentally and emotionally are more complex for the average mental health specialist to understand. The military teaches how emotions can and do jeopardize battle readiness and abilities to conduct battles. They are taught how to suppress these feelings but are never trained in how to reinvest in sharing emotions. When there is no outlet or understanding of how to deal with these suppressed feelings, these veterans are placed in emotional solitary confinement. They have great difficulty in readjusting to civilian life and most can't "turn off" their training from their family life. In many cases, these veterans' marriages succumb to divorce or suicide.

- **Foster children, foster parents, biological parents**—Much has already been shared in the pages of this book; however, each one of these presents a special need for connection with *Unlossable Love*. Each group should have its own focus for treatment or addressing their specific needs; yet, each of these is also interwoven because of how each one impacts the other; for better or worse. So much takes place in these lives which most don't understand. Imagine being the child who is taken suddenly and without any time to say goodbye by child protective services and brought to a complete stranger's home and told they will be staying with them for an undetermined amount of time. Added to this removal, these children are removed from *everything* important to them: their home (physical), their pets, their daily routines, their schools, their friends, and so on. These changes affect each group and present all sorts of issues in adjustments, routines, family structures, structures (or lack thereof), and cultural structures.
- **Mental impairments/illnesses and special needs people**—In this group, one might think that the individual is incapable of understanding emotions and their impacts. This is a misunderstanding on our part: regardless of what might be their diagnosis, every person deserves respect and dignity. A person with special needs or impairments might have limitations to some degree, however, this doesn't give us the right to treat them differently than we

want to be treated and respected. People in this group suffer a great deal because some might not attempt to understand the great potential of love and the *Unlossable Love* **they** can bestow! In all my working with special needs/mental health individuals, I have discovered that when you connect with such individuals in a positive relationship, they thrive and aspire to far greater abilities because someone has taken the time to see them as individuals worthy of not only receiving love but expressing love. To this day, I sometimes see some of my former clients who had moderate to severe impairments. When they see me, they yell and squeal for my attention and will give me a hug or high-five because they are happy to see me. I, in return, show the same excitement because I am happy to see them and their progress. It's such a blessing for all!

I could go on with examples, but you are beginning to see what I mean. We are not equipped to have everything we need for every person as far as having specified training in each area of need. That's okay. The most important thing to equip yourself with is *Unlossable Love* for all people (including yourself). This, with God's leading, will transform more lives than you could ever imagine.

Thank you for reading this book. We hope you have been blessed and encouraged by it and pray for very special blessings to you and yours. May God bless you with His agape/*Unlossable Love* so greatly that it spills over into every aspect of your life. I grant you His peace.